T0324231

Bernard G. Sarnat

20th Century Plastic Surgeon
and Biological Scientist

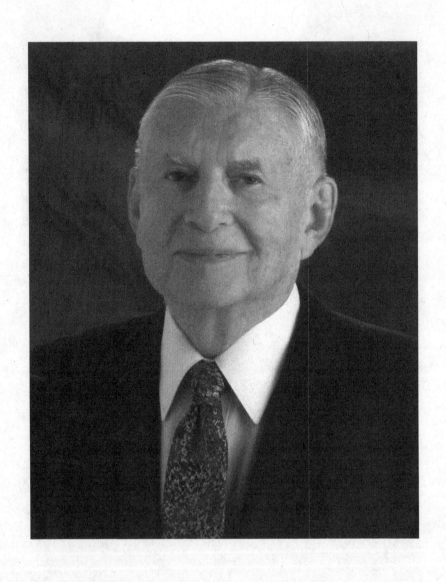

Bernard G. Sarnat

20th Century Plastic Surgeon and Biological Scientist

Pete E. Lestrel

University of California, Los Angeles, USA

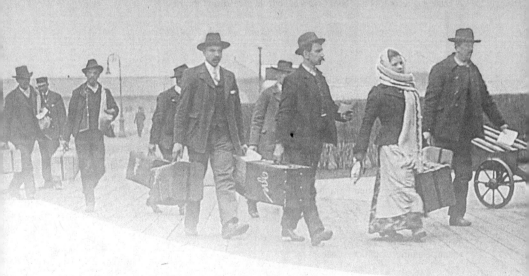

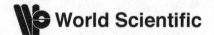 **World Scientific**

NEW JERSEY · LONDON · SINGAPORE · BEIJING · SHANGHAI · HONG KONG · TAIPEI · CHENNAI

Published by

World Scientific Publishing Co. Pte. Ltd.

5 Toh Tuck Link, Singapore 596224

USA office: 27 Warren Street, Suite 401-402, Hackensack, NJ 07601

UK office: 57 Shelton Street, Covent Garden, London WC2H 9HE

Library of Congress Cataloging-in-Publication Data
Lestrel, Pete E.
  Bernard G. Sarnat : 20th century plastic surgeon and biological scientist / Pete E. Lestrel.
    p. ; cm.
  Includes bibliographical references.
  ISBN-13: 978-981-281-317-6 (hardcover : alk. paper)
  ISBN-10: 981-281-317-9 (hardcover : alk. paper)
  1. Sarnat, Bernard G. (Bernard George), 1912- 2. Plastic surgeons--United
States--Biography. I. Title.
  [DNLM: 1. Sarnat, Bernard G. (Bernard George), 1912- 2. Surgery, Plastic
--Biography. 3. Surgery, Plastic--history. 4. History, 20th Century--Biography.
5. Skull--growth & development. WZ 100 S2466L 2008]
  RD27.35.S24 2008
  617.9'5092--dc22
  [B]

                                          2008023231

British Library Cataloguing-in-Publication Data
A catalogue record for this book is available from the British Library.

Copyright © 2008 by World Scientific Publishing Co. Pte. Ltd.

All rights reserved. This book, or parts thereof, may not be reproduced in any form or by any means, electronic or mechanical, including photocopying, recording or any information storage and retrieval system now known or to be invented, without written permission from the Publisher.

For photocopying of material in this volume, please pay a copying fee through the Copyright Clearance Center, Inc., 222 Rosewood Drive, Danvers, MA 01923, USA. In this case permission to photocopy is not required from the publisher.

Typeset by Stallion Press
Email: enquiries@stallionpress.com

Printed in Singapore.

FOREWORD

Fifty years ago, the 600 block of North Maple Drive in Beverly Hills was a remarkable street. My wife, Susie, and I traveled dozens of times the 1,300 miles or so from Omaha in order to visit that particular block. And it was always worth the trip.

What first drew us was the fact that my longtime hero, Ben Graham, had moved there from New York in 1956. Ben had been a huge influence in my life — I named my firstborn son Howard Graham Buffett — and I would have traveled to the ends of the earth at any time to spend a few hours with him.

After Susie and I made our first visit to Ben's new home, we discovered a huge bonus. Across the street lived Ben's cousin, Rhoda Gerard Sarnat, a woman whose extraordinary warmth and intelligence was matched by that of Bernie, her husband. The Sarnats became close friends of ours, a friendship that deepened with every passing year.

The story of the Sarnat and Gerard families is the story of America. Almost immediately, these two bands of immigrants — in a strange land but armed with brains and character — became huge contributors to the wellbeing of their adopted country. This book lets you walk their path, as Bernie Sarnat rises to the top of his profession. Bernie has not only helped thousands of patients to regain a positive self-image and to function better in society, but he has also taught countless students how to be better doctors, thereby multiplying the benefits to society that flow from his talents.

Enjoy a vicarious trip with Bernie through life as I have enjoyed the actual experience.

Warren Buffett

FOREWORD

Dr. Bernard Sarnat (Bernie) has sparkled all his life bringing a glow of living to everyone he has touched. As a surgeon-scientist grounded in medicine, dentistry, general surgery and plastic surgery, Bernie has been an outstanding faculty teacher in Medical Schools and Dental Schools in Chicago, St. Louis and Los Angeles.

Before World War II, plastic surgery was not in the mainstream of surgery. Plastic surgery then consisted of a few esteemed surgeons scattered around the country. After World War II, Bernie and I were among the few founding members of the Plastic Surgery Research Council organized by Drs. Milton Edgerton and Robin Anderson in 1955. We succeeded in directing our clinical and research activities of plastic surgery in the fields of wound healing, burn care, microsurgery, transplantation, cranofacial biology, cranofacial surgery and cancer care.

Dr Sarnat first published on teeth and dental structures. In experimental animals, he used gophers with the vital stain alizarin and demonstrated a 65% decrease in dentin apposition during periods of hibernation. Subsequently, he wrote extensively on the hypoplasia, growth and development of teeth. His study in dogs on the effect on blood circulation of the new drug heparin demonstrated his innate curiosity; he became so engrossed that he even considered pursuing a Ph.D. in physiology. However, he expanded his interest in the metabolism of bones and teeth. These studies ultimately became major contributions during the decades of the development of craniofacial surgery in the last fifty years.

During his career, Dr. Sarnat has been recognized as a caring, skillful and compassionate plastic surgeon. He has been well described as the "Dean of Plastic Surgery" by his Los Angeles colleague, Harvey Zarem, M.D. formerly Chairman of the Division of Plastic and Reconstructive Surgery at the UCLA School of Medicine. It has been a privilege for me to share my surgical life with Bernie for over half a century.

Joseph E. Murray, M.D., F.A.C.S.
Nobel Laureate in Physiology or Medicine 1990

FOREWORD

Atque inter silvas Academi quarere verum. And seek the truth in
the groves of Academy.

(Horace II, ii, 45. 65–8 B.C.E.)

It is with great pleasure that I am privileged and honored to have
been invited to pen a paean to a foreword for my esteemed and
much admired colleague, Bernie Sarnat's biography. Our paths
crossed because of our mutual interests in craniofacial biology, and
our memberships and executive posts in the Craniofacial Biology
Group of the International Association for Dental Research. To
have reached the venerable age of 95 years and still continuing
one's career of seeking truth in the groves of the Academy is indeed
a remarkable achievement. Bernie has been an inspiration to three
generations of students by his critical faculty, his vigor and
thought-provoking ideas and his quiet but dynamic approach.

Bernie helped to change craniofacial biology from a purely
descriptive science into one of experimental and causal analysis. His
long career has bridged profound changes in his chosen field of

craniofacial surgery, transitioning from the era of the lancet and scalpel to the robotic-controlled laser lysing of tissues. Diagnoses have mutated from auscultation, palpation and radiology to CAT-scanning, MRI imaging, ultrasonography and genetically-based prognoses.

In pursuing the biology of the craniofacial complex, Bernie Sarnat followed the footsteps of John Belchier (1736), who fed pigs a madder (alizarin) containing diet to reveal the remodeling of bone by the deposition and resorption of the pink stained bone studied after the sacrifice of the pigs. His study of the developmental approach to the craniofacies provided insights into anatomical variations and congenital malformations, no less than of normal anatomy. Thereby, one could fathom developmental differences from the normal pathways.

My reading of the historical background to this biography provided evidence of the remarkable ethno-cultural traits that preceded and persisted and procreated the apparently inbred characteristics of curiosity, of learning, of questioning that were exemplified in Bernie's life. His life story is in line with the remarkable scientific and cultural community that fled Europe to flourish in the United States. There is an undoubted culturally inherited, hereditary and therefore genetic predisposition to an inquiring mind. The challenge in the current era of molecular biology and genetics is to identify and cultivate these invaluable genes, in contrast to those so tragically inherited by Ashkenazi Jews for their predisposition to Tay-Sachs and Gaucher's diseases. The era of 20th century medicine of post-hoc diagnosis is being replaced by predictive prognoses.

As a student, I recollect vividly my study of Bernie's classical textbook, *The Temporomandibular Joint*, in 1956 that lit my curiosity for craniofacial biology. To have been appointed as a distinguished Bernard G. Sarnat Lecturer in Craniofacial Bone Biology 50 years later was an unimaginable honor that exalted my esteem of his accomplishments.

The generous nature of Bernie is exemplified in the eponymous endowed lectureships in his name in Bone Biology and the

Cedars-Sinai Lectures, and in the Bernard G. Sarnat Prize in the Craniofacial Biology Group of the International Association for Dental Research that is awarded each year to the best student presentation at the annual IADR Meeting.

A "Scholar.Google" search of Bernie's publications reveals some 410 citations, attesting to his prolific productivity and seminal contributions to craniofacial, and indeed to all, biology. He distinguished himself by his unbounded curiosity, unparalleled scholarship, inspirational leadership, modesty and humanity. Bernie's achievements and published works, honored by numerous awards and appointments were broad and will be lastingly influential. He is a scholar's scholar. His combination of knowledge, vision and generosity is epitomized in the biography that follows.

**Geoffrey H. Sperber B.Sc. (Hons),
B.D.S., M.S., Ph.D., F.I.C.D.,
Dr. Med. Dent. (hc).**

CONTENTS

PREFACE

This volume is more than just a biography of a remarkable physician and biological scientist who lived to see most of the 20th century. It is also a story of 20th century America (see Chronology). This is an account that parallels the emergence of America as a world power. While the 20th century was a period of unparalleled scientific accomplishments and technological inventions, it was also one of the most barbarous ones given the Jewish holocaust. Yet America was also a shining beacon attracting immigrants largely from Europe. This is an account of how one immigrant family, with hard work, attained success against considerable odds. It is a narrative of a child born in Chicago to immigrant parents of modest means from Eastern Europe. It delineates the struggle of being a Jew while trying to achieve his desired twin goals of becoming a plastic surgeon and a biological scientist.

Dr. Bernard Sarnat, or Bernie to his friends, is a world famous plastic surgeon and research scientist from Beverly Hills, California. He retired from surgical practice in 1991. However, at the same time that he was active in his practice of plastic surgery, he was also an internationally known biological researcher with appointments in the UCLA Schools of Dentistry and Medicine.

Bernard G. Sarnat S.B., M.D., M.S., D.D.S., F.A.C.S., was born in 1912 in Chicago, a child of immigrant parents from Belarus, Russia, where his two older siblings were born. He was raised on the Northwest side, a predominantly Jewish neighborhood and on the Southside of a largely Protestant/Catholic section of Chicago.

He was an honor student in grammar school and high school and was awarded early admission to the undergraduate college of the University of Chicago with advanced college credit for a number of high school courses. At the end of his junior year he took an undergraduate honors research course in physiology and did exceptionally well. Although his goal was to subsequently obtain a dental degree and specialize in oral and plastic surgery, a result of the influence of his older brother, a dentist, he seriously considered obtaining a Ph.D. in physiology. However, he continued to pursue his studies in medicine. His grades were probably somewhat above average in college but adequate enough to be admitted to the University of Chicago School of Medicine.

During his first six years as a University of Chicago student, this being the years of the Great Depression of the 1930's, it was necessary for him to work in his father's drugstore just off the University of Chicago campus 30 hours a week to make ends meet. He asked to be relieved from work in the drugstore during his seventh and last year in medical school to be able to devote full-time to his studies.

After graduation from Medical School he took an internship at the Los Angeles County General Hospital. He stayed long enough in Los Angeles to take and pass the California Medical State Board examination. He then returned to Chicago and enrolled in the University of Illinois College of Dentistry and graduate school, to conduct research under Dr. Issac Schour. At this time he was also appointed as a junior faculty member. After three years of highly intensive work, Bernie was awarded M.S. and D.D.S. degrees in 1940. In particular, the three years with Dr. Schour were very important formative years for Bernie and provided the basis for serious research programs over the next 60 or more years. Thus, those three years played a major influence for the rest of his life.

Research projects were initiated not only at the University of Illinois but also at the Rush Medical College and the University of Chicago. Significant research of major public health aspects in the relationship of teeth to systemic disease resulted in him receiving a major prize from the Institute of Medicine of Chicago, the first of numerous ones he received throughout his career.

In pursuing his goal of becoming a plastic surgeon he devoted one year as a resident at Cook County Hospital in oral and plastic surgery and a subsequent year in general surgery at University Hospital, also in Chicago. This was followed by another three very busy years learning the art and science of general plastic and reconstructive surgery in St. Louis as a full-time assistant to the internationally famous doctors Vilnay P. Blair and Louis T. Byars.

Bernie's clinical appointments were not only in the private practice office but also in the Department of Surgery at Washington University School of Medicine and Barnes Hospital. Subsequently, he was appointed full professor and head of the Department of Oral and Plastic surgery at St. Louis University School of Dentistry. After three further important developmental years, Bernie returned to Chicago and established his private practice of plastic and reconstructive surgery. At this time he also became professor and Head of the then Department of Oral and Plastic Surgery in the College of Dentistry and also a professor in Plastic Surgery in the Medical School and also the Graduate School. He now had the opportunity to further pursue his basic research program and this also included graduate students. In the ensuing 10 years, significant research was carried out in the general field of bone and craniofacial biology. With this research the Department of Oral and Plastic Surgery established both a national and international reputation.

By 1955 Bernie found that as head of the department he was devoting more and more time to administration and less and less to research. Because of this and health factors, he resigned from all his appointments, closed his office of the private practice of plastic and reconstructive surgery and moved the family to Los Angeles in December of 1955 to start life anew.

Bernie now established his home and private practice office in Beverly Hills and continued his research at Cedars-Sinai Medical Center and at UCLA where he was on the faculties of both the medical and dental schools.

Bernie has more than 220 scientific articles in refereed journals, books and chapters in books. He has lectured extensively, locally, nationally and internationally at many universities and professional societies. As a result he has received more than 25 local, national and international honorary awards.

The author first met Bernie in 1976 when they were colleagues in the section of orthodontics, UCLA School of Dentistry. There the author was exposed to Bernie's broad research interests. This eventually led to a series of joint publications on the shape of the turtle carapace[1,2] and the shape of the rabbit orbit.[3-5] Another aspect of Bernie's considerable abilities not generally known, of which the author has had first-hand experience, has been his organizational abilities as seen at numerous international conferences. His admiration for Bernie has deepened over the years.

In 1987 Bernie received the Distinguished Service Alumni Award from the University Of Chicago Pritzker School Of Medicine and returned for a visit in 1988 (Fig. 48). At that presentation, Thomas Krizek, M.D. Professor and Chairman of the Division of Plastic and Reconstructive Surgery stated the following: "That I should introduce a plastic surgeon from Beverly Hills, California is not a matter of particular surprise; that I should introduce a plastic surgeon-scientist from Beverly Hills sounds more like an oxymoron. Dr. Sarnat, however, is both a distinguished plastic surgeon and a distinguished scientist who, for more than half a century has brought honor to himself, to those of us in Plastic Surgery and to the University of Chicago". Dr. Krizek went on to state that "In 1940 he published his first work on teeth, hypoplasia, growth and development. Forty-seven determined years and more than 200 papers, books, monographs and chapters later. ... That work years ago seemed obscure and without application has now, in the years since..., proved to be without emendation, the basis of what we now understand. He was a scientist in craniofacial surgery when there were no others."

This biography then delineates Bernie's life. It starts with a historical background leading to the emigration of his parents from Belarus to Chicago in 1907, his early childhood years in the 1920's, his formative education, his undergraduate days at the University of Chicago, his graduate degrees received from the University of Illinois and his start in his research career and as a plastic surgeon. In sum, this is a biography of an extraordinary biological scientist and plastic surgeon as well as a warm and affectionate human being. This is then his story.

Finally, I wish to acknowledge my debt to Bernie Sarnat for the many afternoon sessions that extended over some seven years during which I transcribed his recollections and entered them into my laptop. I wish to thank Jascha Hoffman, formerly on the staff of the New York Review of Books, Charles Wolfe and Meredith Bodt for their review of earlier versions of the biography and to Michelle Van Vliet for her photography skills. I also want to thank Hasan Zaidi for his artwork of Figures 1, 2, 4 and 6. Lastly, I owe a debt of gratitude to Sook-Cheng Lim, Scientific Editor at World Scientific Publishing for her guidance during the publishing process. Any errors of omission as well as inaccuracies in interpretation that may have accumulated are solely my own.

Pete E. Lestrel
Van Nuys, California

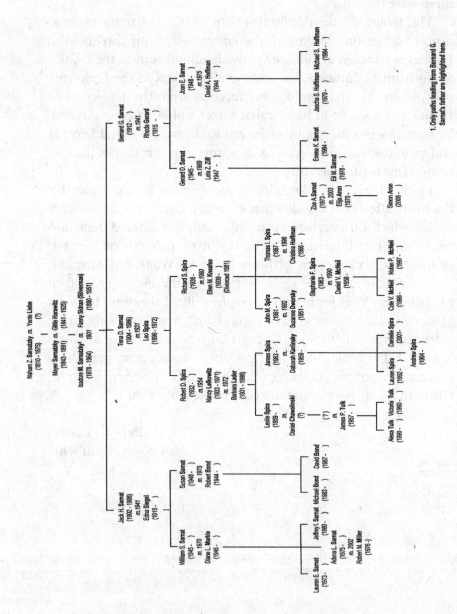

Family Tree of Sarnat

1. Only paths leading from Bernard G.
Sarnat's father are highlighted here.

Part I

BACKGROUND

Chapter 1

BACKGROUND

> If the statistics are right, the Jews constitute but one percent of the
> human race ... His contributions to the world's lists of great names
> in literature, science, art, music, finance, medicine, and abstruse
> learning are also way out of proportion to the weakness of his
> numbers.[1] (Twain, 1899, Vol. 99:535)

In 1907, one Isadore Sarnatzky emigrated from Russia to the
U.S. He was one of the millions of Jewish emigrants to arrive in
New York during the decades from 1881 until the beginning of
World War I. What possible factors could have motivated him to
immigrate to the New World?

In an attempt to understand the reasons that led some of the
Sarnatzky family members, and so many others, to emigrate eventually
to the United States, one must turn to the social, economic and political events that shaped the history of Europe in general, and Russia in
particular, for the 19th and 20th centuries. Without an understanding
and appreciation of that history, it is difficult to comprehend why:
(1) so many Jews left the Old World; (2) so many became highly successful in their newly adopted homelands; and (3) so many bore the
brunt of anti-Semitism[2,3] or more properly anti-Jewishness, in spite of
the fact that their numbers were and remain comparatively few.

In an attempt to try to answer some of these questions, this
biography begins with a look at the historical background. It will

be, of necessity, only a brief sketch, intended to simply introduce the reader to the environment out of which the Sarnatzky family came. It is not intended as a detailed analysis of the economic and social conditions that prevailed at that time. Space precludes such an extended discussion and the reader is directed to the bibliography and elsewhere for the voluminous historical literature on the subject.

What then was the social milieu, which spawned such a large number of notable individuals[4,5] of Jewish descent? One only has to mention internationally known names such as Albert Einstein (1879–1955) and Sigmund Freud (1856–1939). It is noteworthy to add that this pattern of Jewish achievement, especially in the United States, continues to the present day (Table 1). Moreover, given that the total Jewish population is only around 12–14 million or less than 1/24 of 1% of the world's population, it is astonishing that of the 700 individuals who have been Nobel Prize recipients, 127 or about 18% have been Jewish.[6] This is a remarkable accomplishment for such a small population that had to endure the worst persecution of any minority in the 20th century.

These individuals, who were to make significant contributions to business, literature, science, medicine, and countless other fields of endeavor, did so mostly *after* they immigrated out of Europe. The lack of any *in-situ* development in Eastern Europe was a consequence of an oppressive Tsarist regime that prohibited most Jews from attending institutions of higher learning and did not permit them to freely practice their professions.

It is to be admitted that social and political conditions, in general, did improve at the end of the 19th into the 20th century, although such improvements were considerably more noticeable in Western Europe than in Eastern Europe. Nevertheless, the fact that they emigrated was an incalculable loss to the countries in which they had initially worked and resided.

This pattern was particularly pronounced in Germany with the rise of Nazism. Jews who had played a significant part in German science and medicine[4] at the turn of the 20th century saw their pre-eminent role in German science dramatically collapse with the rise

Table 1. Selected List of Individuals of Jewish Descent. Recipients of the Nobel Prize are shown with asterisks.

Name	Birth and Location	Death and Location	Profession
Albert Michelson*	1852, Strelno, Prussia	1931, Pasadena, California	Physics
Albert Einstein*	1879, Ulm, Germany	1955, Princeton, New Jersey	Physics
Niels Bohr*	1885, Copenhagen, Denmark	1962, Copenhagen, Denmark	Physics
Leo Szilard	1898, Budapest, Hungary	1964, La Jolla, California	Physics
Georg Cantor	1845, St. Petersburg, Russia	1918, Halle, Germany	Mathematics
Norbert Weiner	1894, Columbia, Missouri, USA	1964, Stockholm, Sweden	Mathematics
John Von Neumann	1903, Budapest, Hungary	1957, Washington DC	Mathematics
Sigmund Freud	1856, Freiberg, Moravia	1939, London, England	Psychology
Paul Ehrlich*	1854, Strehlen, Silesia, Prussia	1915, Bad Homburg, Germany	Biology
Fritz Haber*	1868, Breslau, Silesia, Prussia	1934, Basel, Switzerland	Biology
Otto Warburg*	1883, Freiburg, Germany	1970, West Berlin, Germany	Biology
Otto Meyerhof*	1884, Hanover, Germany	1951, Philadelphia, Pa.	Biology
Hans Krebs*	1900, Hildesheim, Germany	1981, Oxford, England	Biology
Karl Landsteiner*	1868, Vienna, Austria	1943, New York, New York	Medicine
Albert Sabin	1906, Bialystok, Russia	1993, Washington DC	Medicine
Jonas Salk	1914, New York, New York, USA	1995, La Jolla, California	Medicine
Émile Durkheim	1858, Épinal, France	1917, Paris, France	Sociology
Franz Boaz	1858, Minden, Germany	1942, New York, New York	Anthropology
Ernst Cassirer	1845, Breslau, Silesia, Prussia	1945, New York, New York	Philosophy
Edmund Husserl	1859, Prossnitz, Moravia	1938, Freiburg, Germany	Philosophy
Henri Bergson	1859, Paris, France	1941, Paris, France	Philosophy

(*Continued*)

Table 1. (Continued)

Name	Birth and Location	Death and Location	Profession
Franz Kafka	1883, Prague, Bohemia	1924, Kierling, Austria	Philosophy
Ludwig Wittgenstein	1889, Vienna, Austria	1951, Cambridge, England	Philosophy
Arthur Schnitzler	1862, Vienna, Austria	1931, Vienna, Austria	Playwright
Boris Pasternak*	1890, Moscow, Russia	1960, Peredelkino, Russia	Novelist
Felix Mendelssohn	1809, Hamburg, Germany	1847, Leipzig, Germany	Composer
Jacques Offenbach	1819, Cologne, Germany	1880, Paris, France	Composer
Georges Bizet	1838, Paris, France	1875, Bougival, France	Composer
Gustav Mahler	1860, Kaliste, Bohemia	1911, Vienna, Austria	Composer
Arnold Schoenberg	1874, Vienna, Austria	1951, Los Angeles, California	Composer
Leonard Bernstein	1918, Lawrence, Massachusetts,	1990, New York, New York	Composer
Irving Berlin	1888, Mogilyov, Russia	1989, New York, New York	Musician
Ira Gershwin	1896, New York, New York	1983, Beverly Hills, California	Musician
George Gershwin	1898, Brooklyn, New York	1937, Hollywood, California	Musician
Jascha Heifetz	1901, Vilna, Lithuania, Russia	1987, Los Angeles, California	Musician
Nathan Milstein	1903, Odessa, Ukraine, Russia	1990, London, England	Musician
Benny Goodman	1909, Chicago, Illinois	1986, New York, New York	Musician
Camille Pissaro	1830, St. Thomas, Danish West Indies	1903, Paris, France	Artist
Amadeo Modigliani	1884, Livorno, Italy	1920, Paris, France	Artist
Marc Chagall	1887, Vitebsk, Russia	1985, Saint-Paul, France	Artist
Benjamin Disraeli	1804, London, England	1881, London, England	Politician
Georges Clemenceau	1841, Mouilleron-en-Pareds, France	1929, Paris, France	Politician

of Hitler and his anti-Jewish policies to the detriment of Germany as a whole.[7,8,9] Almost six decades have passed since the end of World War II and Germany has yet to approach her former prominence in science and related fields. However, there was at least one significant difference between the experience of the German Jews in contrast to their Polish and Russian cousins. This was that in Germany, prior to Hitler, Jews were generally permitted to feel at home allowing them to assimilate easily into the German cultural environment in contrast to that of Eastern Europe.[10]

In Eastern Europe, Jews were subjected to a pattern of continuous ill treatment by government officials and government policy. It was this state of affairs that influenced the subsequent history of Jewish emigration patterns in Eastern Europe.[11–13] Thus, to understand the immigration of the Sarnatzky family to the United States and eventually to Chicago, one needs to look back at the social and political milieu that formed 19th century Tsarist Russia. This issue is taken up in the next six chapters.

Chapter 2

TSARIST RUSSIA

We begin the brief historical setting with the year 1492, a year more identified in the West with Christopher Columbus (1451–1506) than with the initiation of one of the greatest forced population movements; namely, the expulsion of over 100,000 Jews from the Iberian Peninsula.[1] This diaspora or expulsion of the Jews from Spain and Portugal in 1492 was not the only one, although perhaps the most well known one, of the numerous expulsions over the centuries. The first exclusion of Jews was initiated by Edward I of England in 1290.[2,3] European expulsions commenced in the 13th century and largely ended by the beginning of the 16th century. Most of the evictions led to a pattern of migration largely directed toward the East and South East Europe but also toward North Africa and the Middle East. By the 17th century, there were only two regions that contained large numbers of Jews: These were the Polish-Lithuanian Kingdom and the Ottoman Empire. Apart from these, there were only a comparatively few Jewish inhabitants in some of the German and Italian cities.

Thus, by the middle of the 17th century, there were less than one million Jews worldwide divided roughly equally between Sephardic (Jews from the Iberian Peninsula) and Ashkenazi (Jews from Central and Eastern Europe) according to Ettinger.[3] There also were Jews living in Moslem-dominated lands such as Syria, Iraq, etc. Statistically, one can roughly estimate that the population of Jews in the 1650's was approximately 0.13% of the total world population. This figure has risen to 0.22% by the year 2000 (Britannica, 2001).

Beginnings in Tsarist Russia

By the beginning of the 18th century, the Kingdom of Poland or the Polish-Lithuanian kingdom,[4] was the largest kingdom in Europe (Fig. 1A), and had been a haven for Jews from the 14th century. Jews served the mainly agrarian society made up of peasants and the Polish nobility composed of the upper and middle class gentry who owned estates. They did this by living in villages and towns where they helped manage the estates and sell the estate-owned products to the villages. They also had the right to distill and sell alcoholic beverages. This latter commodity was a major source of income for the estate owners. Thus, Jews were largely dependent on the landowning nobility for their livelihood. In addition, many Jews eked out a living as artisans, although largely excluded from the existing urban guilds, which viewed them as competition.[3,5]

Nevertheless, in spite of persecution of Jews by the clergy, which viewed Jews only a little above the serfs (the most oppressed class in Poland), many towns in eastern Poland became predominantly Jewish villages. The homes of the Jewish residents would be clustered around the village square where their workshops were located. In contrast, the Christian residents lived semi-agricultural lives in the outskirts.[3] Many of these villages eventually became the *shtetl* (*mestechko*) or, in the plural, *shtetlach* of the 19th and 20th centuries. Because of the restrictions imposed on Jews in the East,[6] these villages developed a close-knit and distinctive community, with the social life based on language (Yiddish), religion and common culture of the members. What was to be called the orthodox way of life for Eastern European Jews[7] revolved around the synagogue, the cemetery, the home, and the marketplace. It was a demanding life for the devout Jew, not only because of the abject poverty that was always present, but also because of the need to adhere rigorously to a strict code of laws that governed daily life.[8]

Part of the reason of why these villages or small towns were tolerated and able to expand unhindered, was that the political regime of Poland by this time was undermined by dissention among the various groups vying for power. Since the 16th century, Poland had been largely a republic with an elective monarchy rather than a hereditary one.[9] The presence of an elective monarchy and the introduction of the free veto (*liberum veto*) in the 16th century were, in part, responsible for the decline. A single member of the national parliament or *diet* (*Sejm*), composed exclusively of the landowning nobility, could exercise the veto nullifying the decision-making in the *diet*. As the nobility was largely obsessed with the pursuit of their own selfish interests at the expense of national concerns and the monarchy, this eventually led to anarchy within the government.[9,10] This general weakening of the regime was to have disastrous consequences at the end of the 18th century (Fig. 1B, 1C and 1D). Thus, in eastern Poland, in particular, as there was little in the way of political stability, this led to laxity in enforcement making it easier for Jews to evade restrictions.[3]

Russian Expansion

Peter I also called Peter the Great (reigned 1689–1725) has been considered by many to be the founder of modern Russia. Under Peter I, the Russian Empire began to expand westward and acquire territory. This Muscovite expansion reached its height under Catherine II, Catherine the Great (reigned 1762–1796), and eventually led to the partitioning of Poland and Lithuania among the three powers, Russia, Hapsburg Austria and Prussia. The increasingly weak central governments of the Polish-Lithuanian Kingdom during 1707–1772, as well as an unstable economy, were major factors inviting Russian and Prussian aggression.[11]

Catherine II and Frederick II, also known as Frederick the Great of Prussia, (reigned 1740–1786) conducted secret negotiations leading to a military alliance in 1764. Catherine II also bribed the Polish nobility who were in positions of influence, to insure that Stanislaw Poniatowski, a weak and indecisive leader, would be elected King.[9] Russian troops moved into Poland to insure a "free" election with the result that the election of Stanislaw Poniatowski, now Stanislaw II Augustus, King of Poland, was unanimous. During the reign of Stanislaw II (reigned 1764–1795), the duly elected king and one-time lover of Catherine the Great,[12] Poland was partitioned on three separate occasions: 1772, 1793 and 1795.[9,13–16]

On the pretext of protecting the Orthodox believers in Poland, the First Partition took place in 1772 (Fig. 1B). With the partition, a treaty signed in St. Petersburg, Russia acquired 12.7% of additional land on the eastern border of Poland-Lithuania and about 1.8 million new inhabitants. Hapsburg Austria received 11.8 % of the new lands, which included Galicia and the southern part of Little Poland, with a total of 1.7 million inhabitants. Prussia took 5% of the land of West Prussia but not the city of Danzig (*Gdansk*). As a result Prussia ended up with 416,000 new inhabitants.[10,15]

After the disastrous results of the First Partition, Poland tried to incorporate reforms and a stronger central government. To achieve her ends, Catherine II had imposed a constitution on Poland that limited the power of the King and increased the power of the nobles. However, in the eighteen years since 1772, the Polish nobility and church hierarchy finally recognized the need to be united against their enemies. Consequently, the Poles were finally able to ally themselves temporarily with Prussia, in part because of Russian preoccupations with Turkey.

In 1789, the Poles abrogated the hated Russian constitution. The new constitution with its reforms was presented in 1791 and was widely applauded throughout Europe.[9] It included a return to a hereditary monarchy and the abolition of the *liberum veto*. Catherine II was bitterly opposed but remained passive initially. Shocked at the dismantling of the French monarchy leading to the French Revolution, she was determined to crush the Polish reform movement. The Polish reforms proved to be short-lived. With the Turkish campaign concluded, the Russian army entered

Poland in 1792 in response to a group of reactionary Polish nobles.[9]

Now joined by Prussia, the Russians routed the Poles leading to the Second Partition in January 1793 (Fig. 1C). Poland now unable to rely on Prussian and Austrian support, and with her earlier ally France preoccupied with revolution, had to retreat. Hapsburg Austria did not participate in the Second Partition of Poland-Lithuania.

This time the Russians took most of Lithuania and Western Ukraine with a total population of 3 million. Prussia took Danzig, Thorn and the northern part of Great Poland, closing the corridor that had existed between the eastern and western parts of Prussia, which added a combined 1.1 million inhabitants.[15] In July 1793, Stanislaw II was forced into signing the Partition treaty in Grodno formally surrendering the territories. Poland did not lose much of its own territory to Russia, as most of the Second Partition took the Lithuanian lands acquired in 1386. However, the loss of Great Poland territory to Prussia was felt to be particularly critical in terms of what little was left of national prestige.[9]

The Poles responded in 1794 with a national uprising, led by Tadeusz Kosciuszko, the commander who had fought with General George Washington during the American War of Independence. Faced with the combined Russian, Prussian and Austrian forces, the Poles fought desperately under their local hero Kosciuszko but were finally defeated. Jews also fought bravely with Kosciuszko and most of the members of a Jewish brigade of light cavalry under the command of Berek Joselevitz gave their lives in the defense of Warsaw.[16] This revolt was crushed by the Russians and Prussians. The Third Partition of October 1795 (Fig. 1D), led to Russia obtaining what was left of Lithuania and the Ukraine with 1.2 million inhabitants, as well as the Duchy of Courland.[15] Prussia gained Warsaw[17] and Hapsburg Austria received territory north of Galicia including Cracow.[9]

After 1795, Poland ceased to exist as an independent political entity. Only in 1918 (and until 1939) did Poland re-emerge as the Second Polish Republic after 122 years of Russian dominance.[15]

One of the results of the three partitions was that over a million Jews in the former eastern Poland were now "acquired" by Tsarist Russia. Prior to the end of the 18th century, Jews were not allowed into the interior of the Russian Empire because they were considered the enemies of Orthodox Christianity by the Tsars.[16,18] Now nearly half of all the Jews in the world resided in the Russian empire.

Catherine II was viewed as "liberal" by the West and considered herself to be a follower of the French Enlightenment as advocated by Voltaire, Montesquieu, Diderot and others. She welcomed the French philosopher Diderot to her court as a tutor to her son as well as carried on a fourteen-year correspondence with Voltaire.

Influenced by the ideas of the Enlightenment, she recognized the need to reorganize the existing legal codes, which were in chaos. She decided to replace the existing law with an entirely new code. To do this she summoned a legislative commission and provided it guidance with her own document called *Nakaz* or the *Great Instruction*. The Nakaz was a compilation based on the ideas of Enlightenment (largely based on Montesquieu's *On the Spirit of the Law* and Beccaria's *Of Punishment and Crimes*). It contained little that was original to Catherine II and its major defect was that the ideas presented were not grounded in the Russian experience but came from a totally foreign quarter; that is, from the West. Moreover, these reforms attempted to improve the misery of the life of the serfs, condemned the use of torture and talked about political freedom and equality. In the end, the legislative commission achieved nothing, largely because of the strong resistance of the conservative nobility[19] that depended on serf labor and was totally against the reforms.[9]

While Catherine II was enamored with the ideas of the Enlightenment, there is some question regarding her sincerity since she did not seem to be overly concerned with whether the commission produced results. It is more likely that she wanted to impress the West that Russia was becoming progressive. In reality, she was greatly dependent on the nobility and their demands, as she owed her throne to them. Eventually she renounced her progressive ideas when she felt that her rule was threatened. With the beginnings of the French Revolution in 1789, she became more reactionary and her reign more repressive. She was shaken by the executions of Louis XVI and Marie Antoinette. By the 1790's, the writings of Voltaire and others were suppressed. She may have initially had sympathy for the serfs, but in the end, she was little moved by their needs.[9,20]

Chapter 3

THE PALE OF SETTLEMENT

Although the Russian government realized that it now had a 'Jewish problem'[1] on its hands, little was initially done and from 1772 to 1791, Jews were permitted to live as they had in what had been Poland, although the economic misfortunes of the peasant population tended to be blamed on the Jews.[2] In 1778, the inhabitants of Russia were classified into various categories. Wealthy Jews were registered as merchants and included in the guilds, the remainder classified as Jewish citizens. Their inclusion within the guilds represented the first time that a European government allowed that to occur, which led to increased tension between the Jewish and non-Jewish members within these corporations. In 1782, the government decreed that all Jewish merchants and citizens had to reside in the larger towns and not in the villages. This represented the beginning of the restriction that Jews could not live any longer in villages.[3]

In 1792, Catherine II issued an edict, which offered certain guarantees to Jews regarding their lives and their religious freedom, but at the same time, it continued the repressive restrictions that had been in force under the Polish regime.[4] Thus, this large population continued to be viewed by both the Russian and Polish officials as a hostile group. Rather than attempting to improve the economic conditions of this largely poverty-stricken population, the Russian and Polish governing classes set out to destroy it by means such as forced assimilation.[5]

The Pale of Settlement

The newly acquired region now stretched from the Baltic Sea in the north to the Black Sea in the south, (encompassing parts of modern Poland, Latvia, Lithuania, Belarus and the Ukraine). The region contained some twenty-five *gubernii* (provinces): nine of which were in what was once Poland and sixteen in what was the region formerly occupied by Lithuania, Ukraine, etc.[6,7] The width from west to east of the Pale[8] was about 640 km (400 miles). On the eastern border was Russia proper and on the western border, the kingdoms of Prussia, Hapsburg Austria and the Ottoman Empire (parts of which eventually became Rumania).

Increasing Restrictions

A 1791 restriction prevented Jews from leaving the newly acquired provinces in the western part of the Russian empire.[3] This territory was eventually to be called the Pale of Settlement (Fig. 2).

By 1812, the pattern of the Pale had been established and Jews could not travel or live outside of the Pale without special permission.[11] This policy was intended to protect Russians from Jewish competition and to keep the greater part of the country clear of Jews.[4] The Pale, in fact, had become a large Jewish ghetto,[9] which was to last, more or less intact, until 1917.

However, the borders of the Pale tended to be in flux, expanding and contracting according to the whims of the Tsar in power.

Initially under Tsar Alexander I (reigned 1801–1825), other policies were put into place to deal with the 'Jewish problem'. Alexander I was convinced that conversion to Christianity was the best method to integrate them into Russian society. One way to encourage this path was to grant concessions to the converts. This included the granting of agricultural land and permission to engage in the manufacture of alcohol — a traditional Jewish occupation that had been restricted earlier.[3] However, the 1804 edict called "Statute Concerning the Organization of the Jews" formulated a dual policy of forced assimilation and expulsion from villages to towns to compel Jews into the general stream of economic and cultural life.

As Ettinger has indicated[3]:

> ...the basic aim of preventing 'acts of injustice and interference in the agriculture of inhabitants of those districts which Jews reside' (as expressed in the preamble of the 1804 statute) — namely, the so-called protection of the peasants against Jewish exploitation — remained the declared policy of the Russian Government... (Ettinger, 1976:813).

This 1804 edict determined where Jews could live inside the Pale and what professions they could pursue. Especially damaging was that Jews were now restricted to towns and could not live in the smaller villages or sell alcohol to peasants.[10] This latter decree was 'justified' as a means to discourage the widespread drunkenness among the serfs. This destroyed the livelihood of a third of the Jewish population who ran village taverns.[11] Full implementation of the 1804 decrees was temporarily curtailed with the start of the Napoleonic Wars.

Chapter **4**

NAPOLEONIC WARS

Under the Russian empire the discontented Polish nobility were receptive to the nationalist revolutionary message coming out of France via the French Emperor Napoleon I Bonaparte (reigned 1804–1815). Following the Prussian defeat at Jena-Auerstädt (1806) Napoleon entered Polish territory and made his headquarters in Warsaw. The Poles were ecstatic that Napoleon had succeeded in removing the Russian and Prussian governments from much of Poland. Moreover, it was hoped that the Napoleon victories would lead to the re-establishment of the Greater Polish state.[1]

French dominance was assured in 1807 with the defeat of the Russians at Friedland, which led to the Treaty of Tilsit. At that treaty, the disposition of Poland was determined and Napoleon agreed to allow Alexander I, Tsar of Russia, a free hand with respect to Sweden.[2,3] While Alexander I was initially enamored with Napoleon's ideas of conquest, he eventually shifted his allegiance to Prussia and England. The territory taken from Poland by Prussia since the first Partition became the Grand Duchy of Warsaw.[4] Much to the dismay of the Polish nobles, the Duchy was placed firmly under French control, while Russia was forced to recognize the Duchy as an "independent" entity. Napoleon shrewdly played the Polish nationalistic card without giving them the independence they wanted, and Poles remained loyal allies to French objectives until the final defeat of Napoleon.[1]

After Napoleon's retreat from Moscow in 1812, he met defeat at the hands of the Russians in the 1813 campaign of Leipzig, which signaled the beginning of the end. The combined might of the Russians, Prussians, Hapsburg Austrians and the English led to the collapse of the French Empire within two years. The victorious allied armies were led into France by Alexander I forcing Napoleon's abdication in 1814 but it took the combined British and Prussians armies to defeat the Napoleonic forces at the final battle of Waterloo in 1815.[3,5]

At the 1815 Congress of Vienna, the victorious powers attempted to re-draw the map of Europe to their advantage. The major purpose of the participants at the Congress of Vienna was to insure that the old hereditary autocratic monarchies were re-established. Also, that any lingering of liberal democratic ideas (such as those that had led to the French Revolution) were stamped out. Post-1815 Europe became politically conservative, bent on maintaining the old order. Ideas such as constitutional government, freedom of the individual and the press, were viewed with suspicion. The idea of equal rights for minorities such as the Jews (termed Jewish emancipation) was viewed as a revolutionary threat to the social order. It took another five decades before emancipation of Jews gradually became a reality in the West. By the 1870's, most of the western monarchies had begun to confer full rights on Jews. Only in Tsarist Russia, would Jews have to wait until 1917.[5]

As a consequence of the congress of Vienna, the Duchy of Warsaw was handed over to Tsar Alexander I as a prize for the Russian efforts in defeating Napoleon. The Duchy was then re-organized into the Kingdom of Poland (also called Congress Poland) with Tsar Alexander I as the hereditary ruler.[1] Initially, to mollify Polish aspirations for independence, the Poles were allowed to maintain a separate government and their own military, albeit controlled by Russian generals. Moreover, they were also allowed to use their own language in carrying out official duties, as well as to maintain Catholicism, so that the existing conditions were not all seemingly negative. However, after 1820, events in Poland became more repressive as Alexander I became more unwilling to abide by the constitution of Poland. He also began to lean more toward the mysticism within the Orthodox Church. One result of these increasingly repressive tendencies of Alexander I was a re-kindling of Polish nationalistic aspirations, which eventually culminated in the failed 1830 Polish Revolution.[1]

The Pale After the Congress of Vienna

By 1820, the Jewish population of the Pale had grown to 1.6 million.[6] By 1825, life in the Pale had become precarious; the majority of settlers lived in poverty. In 1825 Alexander I died to be replaced by his brother Nicholas I.

It was under the tyrannical Tsar Nicholas I (reigned 1825–1855) that the name 'Pale of Settlement' was coined and particularly repressive restrictions such as forced military conscription of Jews was imposed by decree. Nicholas I was not only an absolute autocrat but decided he had to protect Russia from all Western liberal influences and he especially despised Jews.[7] In 1825, a statute decreed that all Jews were to be expelled from a strip 58 km (36 miles) wide along the western border of the Pale joining Russia with Prussia in the north and Austria in the south and forced into the interior of the Pale (Fig. 2). Only towns already containing Jewish communities were exempted at this time.[8] In 1827, restrictions were first imposed on the Jewish residents of Kiev. At that time, Kiev was the largest commercial town in southern Russia.

In 1835, the earlier 1804 statute was reformulated without the clause requiring expulsion from villages, but this did not apply to provinces adjoining the western and especially the eastern borders of the Pale. For example, along the eastern border, Jews were excluded from villages along a strip roughly 240 km (150 miles) in width.[9] This had the effect of further reducing the region available to Jews. In 1843, using this new decree Nicholas I ordered the expulsion of the Jews from Kiev, as well as from the towns of Nikolaev and Sevastopol in the south of the Pale.[8,10,11]

One of the particularly repressive decrees associated with Nicholas I, was the 1827 edict requiring military conscription of Russian Jews. Prior to 1827, Jews were prevented from serving in the military.[12] The idea behind the Cantonist Decrees[13] leading to conscription of Jews, aged 12–25, was forced assimilation; that is, by becoming "Russified" they would influence other Jews upon their return from military service. The period of conscription was set at twenty-five years starting at the age of eighteen for Christians, but Jews could be taken at twelve years of age providing a head start of an extra six years of Russian indoctrination. Conversion attempts in these canton schools to compel acceptance of Christianity were constantly employed, such as forced baptism, and refusal was met with particularly harsh treatment[14] with many dying from the brutal methods.[8] It has been estimated that by 1839 more than 40,000 had been converted to Christianity in Moscow and its vicinity. Few survived the twenty-five years of conscription to return home. Most were never seen again by their families.[10]

The pattern of recruitment was heavily biased toward the poor, unmarried, those who were alone, beggars, unskilled laborers, etc. Moreover, to meet quotas, bands of hunters *khappers* (literally, grabbers) prowled centers of Jewish populations and kidnapped young men without proper papers.[7,10] The policy was highly unpopular.[15] Instead of forced Jewish assimilation, it led to major corruption of the Tsarist bureaucracy via bribery. Jews made every effort to keep their children from being taken into the Russian army.[16] However, avoidance of conscription was not an easy matter. From 1874 to 1892, according to Leeson,[12] 173,434 Jewish recruits were conscripted. Thus, military conscription was clearly one of the reasons driving the extensive Jewish emigration during the last two decades of the 19th century. Jewish migration patterns are taken up subsequently.

In 1850, an edict was passed prohibiting the wearing of Jewish garments but it was difficult to implement. Already in 1848, an edict specifically taxed the wearing of the skullcap. Local officials exploited these regulations to extract payment from Jews.

Probably the harshest measure employed during the reign of Nicholas I was the implementation in 1851 of the proposal to classify the Jews into specific groups to distinguish the minority of "useful" Jews from the "useless" ones. Consequently, according to this "reform program" Jews were categorized into five major groups: merchants, farmers, artisans, permanent townspeople (those who owned property consisting of shops and homes) and town dwellers (i.e., those with non-permanent residences). This last and 'useless' group contained water carriers, wagon drivers, goldsmiths, apprentices, etc. It was this group that was to make up the bulk of army conscription. After 1851, Jews were required to carry documentation that identified their group status. There began a frantic rush to obtain such papers, which led to the use of heavy bribes. Only the Crimean War (1853–1856) and the death of Nicholas I in 1855 prevented full implementation of this so-called "reform" program.[8]

Interestingly, the repressive edicts formulated by Nicolas I did not extend to the far western regions of the Russian empire; namely, into what heretofore had been the kingdom of Poland proper where Jews were the most numerous. Nevertheless, the lot of Jews here was not much better in the face of a rampant and continuous history of Polish anti-Jewishness.[7,10] Eventually by 1914, Warsaw in Russian Poland became the most populous Jewish city in Europe with 350,000 inhabitants. When Poland re-emerged as a political entity (1917–1939) after World War I, the population of Jews had increased to more than three million. By the 1920s, cities with over 50% of Jewish inhabitants included Grodno and Bialystok.[17]

A Momentary Russian Thaw

With the ascent of the liberal Alexander II (reigned 1855–1881), the repressive atmosphere was relaxed with many of the earlier restrictions removed. After thirty years, the repressive 25-year military conscription, including Jewish conscription, was repealed in 1856.

Tsar Alexander II was responsible for the development of the Russian judicial system and more importantly, for the abolition of serfdom in 1861,[18] although in the face of major opposition from the landowners. However, the feeding and education of this large group was another matter.[10,19] A series of decrees between 1859 and 1867 allowed those Jews now considered "useful" to settle outside of the Pale. These included small numbers of doctors and other university graduates as well as merchants, artisans, etc., who were all part of a small developing middle class that tended to be well off and paid high taxes.[10]

Jews now started to participate more in the intellectual and cultural life of the Russian Empire. Moreover, the industrial development of the 1860's following the Crimean War created opportunities for a small group of entrepreneurs in the banking and export trades. Jews also assisted in the building of the Russian railroad system. However, it must be emphasized that these reforms only helped a very small minority; the vast majority of the Jews inhabiting the Pale were probably worse off with little opportunity of earning an adequate livelihood.[8]

A partial survey of 1851 displayed that 91% of the Jews were living in an urban environment and only 3.2% followed agricultural pursuits. This is in stark contrast to the general Russian population, which was 89.3% rural and 6.8% urban.[10]

Thus, the eastern European Jew could not catch up economically with their increasingly prosperous middle class Jewish counterparts in the West, especially in Germany. In fact, by 1871, 60% of all German Jews belonged to the upper middle class.[20] In stark contrast to the economic conditions in Eastern Europe, a 1908 list of the first 200 millionaires in Germany showed that 55 were Jews with economic interests in commerce, finance and banking.[21]

As Ettinger has suggested[8]:

All the spiritual qualities and traits that had evolved throughout the lengthy history of Jewish suffering and vicissitude were now to bear fruit in their capacity for adaptation to new conditions: their intellectualism and respect for learning, their rapid grasp of facts and their analytical ability (Ettinger, 1976:730).

However, this comparative stability and assimilation of German Jews was only temporary and began to change at the end of the 19th century in the face of declining liberalism and the re-appearance of anti-Jewishness.[22] This anti-Jewishness was fueled, in part, by resentment of the cultural assimilation of many Jews and their successful rise into positions of economic, social and even political prominence. Thus, the anti-Jewish propaganda proclaimed that the success of Jews was simply part of an overall campaign to gain control over Christian nations.[8]

The infamous Alfred Dreyfus "affair" clearly mirrored the anti-Jewishness that prevailed in France at the end of the 19th century. Captain Dreyfus, a Jewish French officer was accused of espionage in 1894 in spite of his protestations to the contrary; in 1895 he was found guilty by a secret military court-martial. He was sent to Devil's Island, French Guiana, for incarceration for the rest of his life. An army cover-up, forged documents and Dreyfus's possible innocence led to a vigorous campaign by his supporters and to the famous 1898 open letter "J'accuse!" (I accuse!) by Émile Zola. In 1899 Dreyfus was released from prison and fully exonerated in 1906. Nevertheless, French anti-Jewishness continued to be a force in French far-right politics.

The seeds sowed by this anti-Jewishness in France and Germany, were also to flourish in Eastern Europe.[10] While other factors[23] were also involved, anti-Jewishness was one of the factors that led Germany into World War II.

Although Tsar Alexander II policies seemed liberal at the initiation of his regime, in his later years he also turned reactionary. The reforms, it turned out, had been less motivated by liberalism than by the old aim of increasing Jewish Russification and stimulating commerce and industry in Russia's interior. The vast majority of Jews were not allowed to leave the overcrowded provinces of the Pale.[7] Moreover, there continued to be the long-standing distrust of Jews, a distrust that even Tsar Alexander II exhibited. This essentially precluded the possibility of full civil rights for Jews.[8] Additionally, nationalistic sentiments among Slavs and Ukrainian nationalists were awakening, and with it anti-Jewishness. These groups increasingly attempted to represent the Jews as dangerous opponents of Christianity and thereby opposed to Slavic national aspirations. This ideology tended to emphasize the uniqueness of Russian culture as opposed to the West and Jews were accused of spreading corrupting influences.[8]

Chapter 5

INITIATION OF POGROMS

In 1871, the first major pogrom occurred in Odessa.[1,2] It was stimulated by Greek merchants who were in commercial competition with Jews. The riots lasted for two days and were only stopped on the third day by the police. The government and press hinted that the Jews were at fault, signaling a return to former repressive times. Thus, by the mid 1870's, the mood among many eastern European Jews was one of unease for the future and this premonition of disaster was fulfilled with the murder by revolutionaries[3] of Alexander II, which dashed any hopes for a better life for Jews in Russia.[4,5] In fact, the murder of Alexander II on March 13, 1881, marked the start of the outbreak of pogroms.[2]

Expansion of Pogroms

Shortly thereafter, two rumors started to circulate within the Pale. One indicated that Jews were responsible for the death of the tsar and the other that a *ukase* (edict) was to be passed authorizing people to beat and plunder Jews. Neither rumor had any validity. The government had not singled out Jews or devised any decrees to allow Russians to take revenge for the tsar's murder. However, some in the conservative popular press tended to validate the rumors with their active anti-Jewish campaigns, even before 1881.[2] This was especially the case since some of the papers strongly disapproved of the liberal tendencies toward Jews in Alexander II's government.

In 1881 Alexander III (reigned 1881–1894), son of Alexander II, took the throne and became convinced that Russia had to be purged of all liberal (Western) influences. The assassination of his father reinforced his distrust of liberalism. He resembled his grandfather, the tyrannical Tsar Nicholas I, in maintaining the same narrow prejudicial outlook in regard to Jews.[6] Russian policy now noticeably shifted with the head of the Holy Synod of the Russian Orthodox Church, Konstantin Pobedonostsev (tutor of the young Alexander III), a convinced reactionary who despised the West and its institutions.[7] He generously suggested that one third of Jews should be liquidated, one third forced out by emigration and the remaining third compelled to join the Russian Church.[4]

Within six weeks after Tsar Alexander II's death in 1881, the first pogrom took place in Elizavetgrad; the first one of some 169 recorded ones[8] lasting until 1883. However, pogroms continued well into the 1890's. Several hundred Jews were murdered and many thousands watched their property being destroyed.[4] This first pogrom was initiated by an argument between a Jewish tavern owner and a gentile patron and escalated into a major pogrom with the mob assisted by peasants coming in from an adjacent village anxious to share in the Jewish loot.[2]

These pogroms were condoned, if not organized,[9,10] by the Minister of the Interior, Ignatiev.[5] Nevertheless, the presence of pogroms[11,12] carried out by local initiative caught the government with surprise and eventually led to the removal of Ignatiev. One of the last acts that Ignatiev carried out before his dismissal[13] was the 1882 anti-Jewish legislation called the May Laws,[14] which were then used to justify the pogroms. An identical policy was later followed by the Nazis with the enactment of the Nuremberg Laws of 1935. These regulations severely affected Jews in the Pale who were already faced with a precarious existence due to the overcrowded conditions. The local authorities, in turn, used the May decrees to harass and exploit Jews using blackmail and demands for bribes. Additionally, Ignatiev declared in 1882 that the western border is open to Jews, suggesting that they were free to leave.[12] The effect of these governmentally sanctioned actions (from

1881–1911) was to stimulate the greatest emigration of Jews since the Spanish episode of 1492.

The Pogrom Initiators

Who were those *pogromshchiki* who carried out the pogroms? It has been argued that they were largely unemployed workers from Moscow and St. Petersburg, a consequence of an economic recession present at the time, who traveled in bands along railroads from town to town. They were joined by local townsmen and peasants in the beating and robbing of Jews. It has been shown that the location of the pogroms followed the railroad lines.[10]

In response to the pogroms of 1881, the Jewish leadership, a conservative body, based in St. Petersburg, attempted to deal with the problems by convening a conference (Conference of Jewish Notables) in April of 1882. The conference included around forty of the most prominent Jews in Russia. Of the two alternative solutions on the table, emigration or emancipation, the group opted for emancipation because emigration was costly, impractical, and disloyal as well as against Russian law.[2] Opposed to this view were members of the newly politically active intelligentsia, a group of journalists and writers, who questioned the motives of the St. Petersburg leadership on the grounds that they (the leadership) did not want to endanger their privileged status by supporting a policy (emigration) that was strongly opposed by the government. Moreover, the intelligentsia argued that the policy of emancipation (or assimilation) did little to prevent pogroms.[2] Although, the question of emigration versus emancipation may have been a hot issue for debate in St. Petersburg, for the traumatized inhabitants of the Pale, looking to escape the deteriorating conditions, emigration was viewed as the only way out.

In 1881, thousands of Jews fled across the western border of the Pale to Brody, an overcrowded border town in Hapsburg Austria.[12] With the aid of Jewish organizations, some of these refugees entered the United States, but a majority had to return to their homes in the Pale. Jewish organizations lost control over migration due to the sheer magnitude of the numbers involved. As Ettinger indicated, this led to migration being largely based[12]:

> ...on individual initiative, as family members who had established themselves in the New World brought over their relatives (Ettinger, 1976:861).

This pattern of personal initiative was also very much present in the Sarnatzky family. It fueled their ambitions to succeed and the desire for a better life for themselves and their children (as will be documented in the next Chapters).

Thus, the Pale was now to bear witness to particularly unfortunate and tragic events that shaped Eastern Europe and played a significant role in the new Jewish Diaspora. This Diaspora was to affect the lives of millions of Jews who either left on their own volition for various reasons or were forced to leave by governmental decree. In 1887, new educational restrictions limited the number of Jews attending universities. They were limited to ten percent within the Pale and five percent outside of the Pale. Moscow and St. Petersburg were the exceptions; here the quota was limited to three percent.[6] Restrictions were also placed on the legal profession, and in 1889, it was decreed that no Jew could be called to the bar without permission of the Minister of Justice; few Jews were called.[6]

After 1888, the anti-Jewish campaigns intensified, in part due to the 'miraculous survival' of Tsar Alexander III and his family in a railway accident. This accident was viewed as a sign from above by the conservative Pobedonostsev, head of the Holy Synod of the Russian Orthodox Church.[16]

Toward the end of the last two decades of the 19th century, conditions had deteriorated and most rural areas of the Pale were banned to Jews. Conditions had become so impoverished that about one-third of the Jewish population in the Pale required some kind of economic assistance from Jewish welfare organizations to survive.[15]

The economic plight of Jews in Bessarabia, the most south-western province of the Pale adjoining the Black Sea, was observed by the governor of Bessarabia who commented that[17]:

... The houses along second-rate and even back streets are occupied in unbroken succession by stores big and small, shops of watch-makers, shoe-makers, locksmiths, tinsmiths, tailors, carpenters, and so on. All these workers are huddled together in nooks and lanes amid shocking poverty. They toil hard for a living so scanty that a rusty herring and a slice of onion is considered the tip-top of luxury and prosperity (Cutler, 1996:54).

In addition, in 1891, in a particularly notorious incident, about 20,000 Jews who as artisans had legal residency status in Moscow were now forced out of the capital and into the Pale. These expulsions were carried out by force, some even in chains with police escort. This expulsion order was justified by the Tsarist regime on the need to purify the sacred historical capital.[12] In the same year, another 2,000 were deported from St. Petersburg to the Pale. It is thus, not surprising that these conditions led to the mass emigrations that spanned four decades until the onset of World War I.

Chapter **6**

JEWISH EMIGRATION

Toward the end of the 19th century, Russian governmental attitudes had begun to change with respect to emigration. Emigration was now seen as the solution to an apparently insoluble Jewish problem. The Russian leaders looked forward to the time when at least the larger cites would be empty of Jews.[1]

From 1881 on, out-migration greatly increased, Jews leaving on an average of 50,000 a year. In 1891, over 100,000 had left, and in 1892, this number had increased to 137,000. In spite of this large flow of out-migration, there were still over four million Jews left in the Pale by 1885. According to the census of 1897, there were 5,216,000 Jews living in Russia. Of these, 4,899,300 Jews, comprising 94% of the total Jewish population, lived in the Pale and comprised half of the world's Jewish population. This number represented 11.6% of the total general population of Tsarist Russia and 14% of the population of Russian Poland.[2,3,4] This number increased to over five and a half million by 1914 when the World War I largely stopped emigration.

Russian Policy

Consequently, it could be said that Russian policy of forced emigration was an unmitigated failure since the number of Jews did not dramatically fall with emigration, and actually, the opposite took place. The region of the Pale acted like a reservoir, constantly replenishing the Jewish population[5,6] in spite of the continuous emigration.[7] What the emigration policy did do was to account for the natural population increase and transfer it elsewhere.[8,9] Finally, Jewish emigration was not just confined to the Russian Pale. Jews also emigrated in large numbers from other countries that exhibited repressive governmental policies such as Rumania and Austria.

On a broader scale, by the beginning of the 19th century, the population of Tsarist Russia was overwhelmingly rural with only 4% living in urban communities. This pattern only gradually changed with time. From the middle to the end of the 19th century, the Tsarist regimes felt that the modernization of the agricultural base was probably next to impossible and that the only solution was to introduce industry on a large scale. This would allow the removal of people from the land and into cities and thereby ease the rural poverty among peasants. Consequently, this led to acceptance of capital from the West for the construction of railroads, oil wells and factories. Unfortunately, all this did was to add a poorly paid and ill-fed urban workforce to an already impoverished peasantry. This led to the widespread perception that one worked for the benefit of foreign investors (and some Jews) and the Tsarist autocracy.[10] This was then a social milieu that fed the already prevalent anti-Jewishness and eventually led to the October Revolution of 1917.

The last Tsar, Nicholas II (reign 1894–1917), made no basic changes in regard to governmental policy toward Jews at the beginning of his reign. The lot of those Jews, who had not participated in the out migrations from Eastern Europe, did not materially improve. In fact, conditions had largely worsened. The continuation of Tsar Nicholas II's autocratic rule — especially the lack of expected liberal reforms — eventually initiated fundamental changes in the Russian social milieu leading to the October Revolution of 1917 and the eventual takeover by the Bolsheviks. Opposition to Nicolas II who was clearly anti-Jewish, arose with the realization that the anti-Jewish governmental policies in place were deliberate and aimed at consolidating power and control over the majority of the population, not solely the Jews. Writers such as Maxsim Gorky (1868–1936) and others began to attack the government and speak out against the persecution of the Jews.

From 1884 to 1903, there was a momentary respite from the pogroms, although conditions did not materially improve in the Pale, and emancipation was still a long way off. Emigration however, continued with an average of forty thousand Jews leaving Russia each year.[6] A new movement called Zionism, especially under the leadership of Theodor Herzl gathered momentum and adherents. This movement had advocated wide-scale emigration since the pogroms of 1881 and the establishment of a Jewish State. Also, a radical Jewish workers organization called the Bund, advocated armed physical resistance and self-defense in the struggle for emancipation and civil rights. It advocated, for the first time, a sense of pride, self-awareness and self-confidence. However, because the Jewish community tended to favor the traditional non-violent approach, the Bund was never universally embraced because of its revolutionary aims, although it was favored as a means to defend against the pogroms. The problem was that members of the Bund were viewed as revolutionaries, and this played directly into the anti-Jewish press, which branded all Jews as revolutionaries or enemies of the state; thus, providing the propaganda used for justifying pogroms.[6] As these developments took place in the Jewish community, the pogroms of 1903–1906 started.

Increasing Pogroms

This new round of pogroms, more violent and wide-ranging than the ones of 1881–1883, had their origins initially as isolated incidents, which intensified with the Russo-Japanese War and the 1905 Revolution. Jews again became unwilling scapegoats for the failed policies of the tsarist government.

Consequently, out-migration continued at an unabated pace,[1] fueled by pogroms of 1903–1906. In Kishinev[11] (now Chisinau, Moldavia), a city not far from Odessa near the Black Sea, the pogrom of April 19–21, 1903 was particularly violent[6,12] with 47 Jews murdered, 424 injured, 700 houses burned and 600 shops looted,[13] while the local authorities did nothing to prevent the carnage.[4] This particular pogrom generated worldwide condemnation and prompted the Russian author Leo Tolstoy (1828–1910) to write in a letter[2]:

> ... I fully realized the horror of what had taken place, and experienced simultaneously a burning feeling of pity for the innocent victims of the cruelty of the populace, amazement at the bestiality of all these so-called Christians, revulsion at all those so-called cultural people who instigated the mob and sympathized with its actions... I felt a particular horror for the principal culprit, our government with its clergy, which fosters in the people bestial sentiments and fanaticism, with its horde of murderous officials. The crime committed at Kishinev is nothing but the direct consequence of that propaganda of falsehood and violence which is conducted by the Russian Government with such energy (Cutler, 1996:53)

In addition to Kishinev, pogroms broke out in Smela, Rovno, Sosnowiec, Gomel, and in all twenty-five such towns which suffered pogroms, the authorities again did not attempt to curtail. In September 1904, another twenty-four localities were subjected to pogroms; these were instigated by soldiers waiting to depart for Manchuria to fight in an increasingly ineffective and unpopular war. These pogroms continued until December 1904, encouraged by an anti-Jewish press.[6]

Pogroms became especially severe after the social upheavals caused by the defeat of the Russians at the hands of the Japanese in the 1904–1905 Russo-Japanese War. Jews were made one of the scapegoats responsible for the Russian misfortunes. In particular, the Tsarist regime felt that by focusing attention on Jews it could deflect the criticism of its autocratic rule and thereby affect a new *rapprochement* between the Russian people and the monarchy.[8] This policy was a failure and not only led to increased resistance but also hastened the eventual collapse of the Tsarist regime.

During the summer and autumn of 1905 and continuing until September 1906 when the pogroms ended, Jews were attacked in 657 pogroms. In Bialystok and Odessa, hundreds were killed and thousands injured while police stood idly by. The total count was 3,103 killed and tens of thousands injured in a year and a half of rioting.[14] What is not evident from these statistics is the extent of the excessive violence and atrocities carried out by the *pogromshchiki* who in many ways represented Russian society in 1905.[6] Also, for the first time, the government was directly implicated in the attacks on Jews. These pogroms triggered a new round of emigrations, which temporarily ceased with the onset of World War I.[1,4,8]

After the 1905 Revolution, and fortunately for the residents of the Pale, the tsarist government finally moved in and re-established control, discouraging all demonstrations and pogroms. Nicholas II had recognized that popular demonstrations, whether reactionary or revolutionary, could be equally dangerous.[6] However, this re-establishment of order was only to last until 1917.

Shtetl towns such as Piesk (Peski) and Mosti suffered intensified Jewish oppression because many of the Jewish residents had participated in the abortive uprisings of 1905 to overthrow the hated Tsar Nicholas II.[15] The town of Piesk, as countless other towns in the Pale, was similar to Skidel,[16] the town from which the Sarnatzky family emigrated. Thus, it seems likely that these pogroms influenced Bernie's father, Isadore Sarnatzky, among others of the Sarnatzky family, to seek a way out and emigrate from Tsarist Russia.

Initially, leaving Russia was illegal and required large-scale bribes to border officials. It was only after 1907 that emigration was legalized and passports easier to obtain.[4]

Emigration routes from 1881 to 1914 for Jews from the Pale included land routes such as Brody and Cracow in Austria–Hungary, but the majority left via sea routes from areas in the north containing towns like Riga, Libava, Danzig, etc., and from towns in the south like Odessa and Sevastopol.[17]

In the pogrom years of 1905–1906, over 200,000 Jews left Russia. From 1881 on until the outbreak of World War I, Jews left Eastern Europe for Australia, Canada, Great Britain, Palestine, South Africa, South America, United States and other parts of Western Europe.

Some of distinguishing features of the Jewish migration patterns were that: (1) the number of children was twice the average of other immigrant groups, (2) only about 6% of Jews returned to their countries of origin as compared with a third among other immigrants; and (3) nearly half of these eastern European Jewish immigrants had no defined occupation (i.e., no permanent source of livelihood) in contrast to 25% of other immigrant groups.[8]

From a demographic perspective, dramatic changes occurred especially from 1875 onwards. Jewish population worldwide was 7.5 million at the beginning of the 1880's, increasing to 11 million by 1900 and rising to more than 16.5 million by the eve of World War II.[8] Jews had become largely urbanized by World War I. At the beginning of the 19th century, they had been overwhelmingly village and town dwellers, now they resided in the large metropolitan centers of the world.[4]

Chapter 7

THE BOLSHEVIK REVOLUTION

After the collapse of Russia in the October Revolution of 1917, the provisional government led by Alexander Kerensky was warmly greeted by Jews since it abolished all limitations based on religion or nationality and granted equal rights. Unfortunately, it proved to be short-lived, lasting just seven months. In the Ukraine, the 1917–1920 battles between the Red Russian (Bolsheviks[1,2]) and various White Russian armies[3,4] vying for control of the Soviet regime, led to the worst pogroms of the 20th century in which many innocent Jews lost their lives.[4-6]

Communist Takeover

Utilizing the ideas developed by Karl Marx (1818–1883), an ardent anti-religionist as well as anti-Jewish, of an economic class struggle between the bourgeois and the proletariat,[7] in which the proletariat would be ultimately victorious, formed the ideology behind what became the successful communist takeover of the Russian regime. A troika composed of Lenin (1870–1924; held power 1918–1924), Leon Trotsky[8] (1879–1940) and Joseph Stalin (1879–1953; held undisputed power from 1928–1953), also anti-Jewish, led the Bolshevik takeover in 1918. However, complete control over their Civil War opponents did not take place until 1922. Trotsky played an essential part in leading the Red army, and without his energetic leadership, the Bolshevik revolution might never have succeeded. Nevertheless, Trotsky as a

Jew from Odessa was alienated from Judaism as were many other secular Jewish Bolsheviks, resulting in his behavior being anti-Jewish.[9]

Lenin, a non-Jew,[10] claimed to be against anti-Jewishness, declaring that it had no place in a 'classless' society, even though he did not necessarily either accept Jewish culture or the idea of a national Jewish identity (especially Zionism). Lenin wrote in the margin of a 1917 decree condemning anti-Jewishness that[4]:

> "*Pogromchiks* and those that carry on pogrom agitation are to be considered outside the law" (Sachar, 1953:383).

As far as he was concerned, Jews did not constitute a separate cultural group since that ran against the idea of the Jewish proletariat, as everyone was equal under the communist regime. Anti-Jewishness (however not Zionism) was now temporarily reduced as it was viewed as a counter-revolutionary activity by the regime. In theory, if not always in practice, Jews were to be treated equally like all other groups under the Russian communist ideology.[4] Thus, not unlike the earlier Tsarist regimes, the Bolshevik approach was that given equal rights, Jews would rapidly assimilate; the regime was to be sorely disappointed.

Under Lenin's terrorist campaign intended to insure absolute control, certain groups were earmarked as members of an antisocial group. Besides the Zionists, groups such as Jewish traders became one of the categories, making them class enemies open to persecution and possible arrest. Jews learned to fear the communist regime in the same way they did the Tsarist regime of earlier times.[9]

Religious groups, especially, were driven underground, as Marxism had no place for them. Thus, the condition of religious Jews (in contrast to secular ones) in Russia deteriorated after the replacement of the provisional Kerensky government by the Bolsheviks[9]:

> In August 1919, all Jewish religious communities were dissolved, their property confiscated and the overwhelming majority of

synagogues shut forever. The study of Hebrew and the publication of secular works in Hebrew were banned (Johnson, 1987:453).

By 1920, Zionism began to be viewed as a threat by the regime. As one of a number of democratically organized structures, labeled as a bourgeois institution, it was suppressed. Consequently, many Zionists found themselves incarcerated and sent to Siberian camps set up by the new regime.[11]

By 1922, the Union of Soviet Socialistic Republics (USSR) had been established and by 1925, the USSR had become an increasingly oppressive dictatorship ruled by the Russian Communist party. With communism all economic resources were controlled by the state, private property disappeared; capitalist enterprises and economic competition became illegal. Given these economic policies, millions of Russians were reduced to poverty, Jews among them.[4]

Improving Social Conditions

However, Jews could now move out of the Pale of Settlement, and many did, moving from the villages to the larger cities like Moscow, Leningrad, Odessa, Kiev and Kharkov. Many of these moves by unemployed Jews were triggered by disasters, such as the savage pogroms in the Ukraine (1918–1920) and the worsening economic conditions, which led to widespread famine (1920–1921) and virtually ended the village or *shtetl* way of life in regions of the former Pale.[11]

To ameliorate the economic conditions, the development of Jewish collective farms starting in 1925 eventually led to the re-settlement of more than 225,000 individuals to the southern Ukraine and Crimea. By 1930, fully 10.1% of Russian Jews were now involved in agriculture. In 1927–1928, Jews were also settled in Birobidzhan, a remote area in eastern Siberia near the Chinese border, but this experiment was less than successful because of the severe climate.[4,11]

Eventually the revolutionary changes took hold and gradually the lot, especially for the younger secular Jews, improved. As secular Jews, with their commercial and administrative skills well above the Russian average, they became disproportionably represented in the higher ranks of the Communist Party apparatus. Educational opportunities also increased, including previously unattainable professorships and memberships in scientific academies.

With Stalin's rise to power, pressure on Jews increased and all forms of Jewish religious activity and cultural expression were largely destroyed by the late 1920's.[9] Moreover, with the onset of the Stalinist purges in the mid to late 1930's, the lot for all Jews as well as Russians in general, began to deteriorate. Thousands of intellectuals, Jews among them, were sent to the *Gulags,* or corrective labor camps.[4]

Anti-Jewishness temporarily diminished in Russia during the so-called "Great Patriotic War" as Stalin appealed for help from all Russians and roughly half a million Jews fought for the Red Army. But the improvement was not to last. During the last years of the Stalinist regime, and with governmental approval, the old hatreds of Jews again resurfaced.[12] From 1948 to 1953, as a matter of state policy, Jews were systematically prevented from employment in governmental positions, trade associations, research institutes, universities, military academies, etc., a move which was, an immeasurable loss to the communist regime and painfully reminiscent of Nazi Germany. In addition, more and more Soviets, including Jews, disappeared or were sent to the *Gulags* as Stalin's paranoia increased. By 1952, virtually the entire leadership of Soviet Jewry had been eliminated via show trials that found them guilty of totally bogus charges of treason. Conditions improved only after Stalin's death in 1953.[4]

It is ironic that for many centuries, Jews were not allowed *into* the Russian empire while between the 1950's and 1980's, Jews were not allowed to *leave*.[13] This Russian policy against Jewish emigration was only ameliorated after the policy of glasnost (openness) was advocated by Mikhail Gorbachev (1931–) and leading to the eventual collapse of the USSR.

In contrast, most of these rights (those available to Soviet Jews) were generally not attainable to any degree from the beginning of the newly constituted Polish national state[14] created out of the western part of the Pale. Rampant anti-Jewishness remained the rule, a pattern that has continued well into the 1990's. Lech Walesa (1943–) former leader of the Solidarity Movement has apologized for anti-Jewish actions, but there remains ambiguity about the sincerity of other Polish leaders.[4,6,15]

Chapter 8

EMIGRATION TO THE UNITED STATES

E migration of German Jews to the United States first took place in the early part of the 19th century. They were among the earliest Jewish settlers to emigrate and were well established in the United States before the large migrations of the later part of the 19th century. Subsequently, from 1881 to 1914, about 2.4 to 2.75 million Jews left Eastern Europe (largely from the Pale but not totally limited to that region) for other parts of the world. Around 80% of these Jewish emigrants went to the United States. These Jewish immigrants constituted about 9–10% of the roughly 22 million European immigrants that were to make a new life in the United States.[1,2]

Emigration Trends

With over 2 million Jewish inhabitants in the United States by 1900 and 2.5 million by 1914, the Jewish community became a factor in American cities. Of these immigrants, the vast majority was poor and had no knowledge of either the English language or the culture of the country that was to become their new home. The overwhelming majority of Jewish immigrants settled in the larger cities on the Eastern seaboard. The social need to live near relatives initially led to overcrowding in Jewish areas of residence. Since Jewish immigrants from areas such as the Pale were largely penniless on arrival, they entered at the bottom of the immigrant social ladder.[3]

Initially, Jewish immigrants entered the workforce either as manual laborers or as peddlers offering their goods for sale from door to door. Many of the immigrants were absorbed into the garment industry (wholesale tailoring) because many of them had been employed in that occupation in Eastern Europe. This led to the rise of sweatshops with workers doing piecework at low wages. It was in response to these onerous working conditions that the first Jewish trade unions arose. A catalyst for the union movement was the New York Triangle Shirtwaist Company fire of 1911 in which 146 immigrant women lost their lives. The organization of labor eventually led to an increase in the standard of living as well as higher income levels which allowed them to bring their relatives to the United States as well as provide financial aid to those still living under repressive conditions in Eastern Europe.[3]

Between the 1840's and the 1860's, a Jewish community was established in Chicago. By 1852, there were about two hundred Jews. By 1860, this number had increased to 1,500 out of a total population of 112,000.[4] These Jews were largely of German descent, and although some Polish-Russian Jews had also arrived in Chicago, the large influx of Eastern European Jewry was yet to come (Fig. 3).

By 1900, the 20,000 German Jews were outnumbered by the 50,000 Eastern European Jews.[4] The relationship between the earlier, and now largely assimilated German Jews, and their Eastern European brethren who arrived later, was anything but cordial. The former group, speaking German, now middle class, successful in business enterprises and practicing Reform Judaism, was viewed as German rather than Jews. In contrast, the largely poverty-stricken, recently arrived, Eastern European Jews tended to bring their *shtetl* traditions with them to Chicago. They wore traditional clothes and practiced Orthodox Judaism. Few could read or write English. While German Jews were embarrassed by these Old World ways, they were more concerned that these Eastern European Jews might set off anti-Jewishness, which the German Jews had managed to largely diffuse over the years. They were apprehensive that the amiable relationships built over the years with gentiles might be threatened.[4] In the words of Bernard Horwich, who had arrived in Chicago from Eastern Europe in 1880[4]:

> The attitude of the German Jews toward their Russian and Polish brothers was one of superiority and unpleasant pity. They tolerated them only because they were Jews, and one would often hear the German Jews bewailing their fate — that they, Americanized businessmen, had to be classed in the same category with the poor, ignorant, ragged Jewish peddlers on the other side of the river, on Canal Street (Cutler, 1996:95).

Consequently, German Jews embarked on extensive programs to help the newcomers assimilate into American society. This was accomplished by financial, educational, and other social-service institutions. This was done not only out of sympathy for their plight but also for self-protective reasons. The Eastern European Jews tended to view this assistance with some suspicion initially as they tended to rely on assistance within their own group, as they had done in the Old World. Moreover, there was the issue of language since the German Jews did not either speak or understand Yiddish, the language of the *shtetl*. Socially, the two groups tended to remain separate.[4]

Between 1880 and 1910, the region on the Near West Side of Chicago became known as the "Poor Jews Quarter" and later as the Maxwell Street area. The crowded area was composed of over fifty-five thousand largely poor East European Jews.[4] Sections of the Maxwell Street area or "Jew town" as it was known resembled a transplanted East European *shtetl*. It was viewed as an exotic Old World market area to be visited by Jewish and non-Jewish onlookers alike. Bernie recalled his mother taking him there as a child to see how the people lived and bargained for goods. The last remains of what was once a vibrant Jewish area were bulldozed by the city in 1994 and the land sold to the University of Illinois at Chicago.[4]

Gradually however, Jewish immigrants adapted to their new cultural environment. Many second-generation immigrants went to college, which in turn allowed increased access to white-collar professions. Eventually this urban concentration in large cities had two contradictory effects: a weakening of the influence of tradition leading to increased cultural assimilation and a strengthened sense of solidarity within the Jewish community.[3]

Recent Population Trends

Based on 2005 figures, countries with over a quarter million Jews include the United States with 5,652,000, making it the country with the largest number of individuals of Jewish ancestry, with Israel coming in second with 5,235,000. At that time, France was third with 494,000, Canada with 372,000 was fourth, the United Kingdom was fifth with 298,000, while the Russian Federation with 235,000 was sixth (Table 2).

In spite of the attention that Jews have received over the centuries, they have never represented a large population when viewed from a worldwide perspective. The figures for the year 2000 and 2005 demonstrate that Jews only account for a little more than 0.2% of the world's population. Moreover, the total Jewish population is beginning to show consistent decreases from 1984 to 2005, reflecting a pattern of population loss increasingly displayed by many first world nations.

Over the last six decades, substantial demographic changes have affected Jewish population numbers. Jews in the United States are now estimated at 5,652,000, a slight loss from 1984 numbers. Israeli population figures have substantially increased to 5,235,000, mostly due to immigration from Russia and elsewhere. Figures for the former USSR show major losses since 1984. These are due to emigration with approximately 235,000 Jews remaining in 2005. The Jewish population of France is estimated at 494,000 and the United Kingdom at 298,000, one displaying a loss since 1984 and the other a slight gain. The population of Canada is now estimated at 372,000, showing an increase since 1984. Finally, the total world Jewish population as of 2005 is estimated at 13,033,000. Note that this figure is still 20% less than the estimated 16.6+ million (1939)

Table 2. Jewish Population Estimates (1939–2000). Countries Ranked Containing More Than 1% Jews as a function of the total Jewish World Population.

	1939[a]	1984[b]	2000[c]	2005[d]	% of Jewish Population
United States	4,770,000	5,720,000	5,700,000	5,652,000	43.4
Israel	449,000	3,380,000	4,882,000	5,235,000	40.2
USSR[e]	3,200,000	1,760,000	438,100	235,000	1.8
France	320,000	670,000	521,000	494,000	3.8
Canada	155,000	310,000	362,000	372,000	2.9
United Kingdom	340,000	360,000	276,000	298,000	2.3
Argentina	220,000	250,000	200,000	185,000	1.4
World Totals	16,648,000	13,370,950	13,191,500	13,033,000	~0.2

a. Year 1939 estimates are from various sources.
b. Year 1984 estimates are from Sachar (1985).
c. Year 2000 estimates are from DellaPergola (2000).
d. Figures for 2000, 2005 refer to the Russian Federation, not the USSR.
e. The Jewish People Policy Planning Institute (2005)
Note: Considerable caution should be exercised in the interpretation of these population estimates because they tend to vary substantially from source to source. They should be treated as rough estimates only.

on the eve of World War II, reflecting the substantial effect of the Holocaust.

With this material as background, we are in a better position to understand why so many families left the Old World in general, and why numerous members of the Sarnatzky family, in particular, chose to immigrate to the United States. The exact motivations that prompted individuals such as Isadore Sarnatzky to leave the Old World remain uncertain and open to interpretation. Nevertheless, one can suggest a number of factors that may have influenced the decision-making. First may have been the unstable political situation and numerous pogroms. Friends and acquaintances that had emigrated may have written letters urging them to follow. Other reasons might have included the usual lack of educational opportunity for one's children, the limited economic conditions, lack of suitable spouses, avoidance of military conscription, and, finally, a thirst for adventure in a different land.

The next chapters take up the story of what took place when some of the members of the Sarnatzky family found themselves in a new and strange country called the United States of America.

Chapter 9

A NEW CENTURY

The United States at the turn of the 20th century was a very different place especially when viewed from the vantage point of the beginning of the 21st century. The United States consisted of 45 states. Arizona, New Mexico and Oklahoma, along with Alaska and Hawaii, had not yet joined the union. The years prior to World War I were ones of unbridled optimism for most Americans, who took their cue from President Theodore Roosevelt (1858–1919; President: 1901–1909). He embodied this new found optimism and self confidence, in spite of political corruption, child labor, widespread slums in the cities, high mortality from pneumonia, malaria, diphtheria, typhoid fever, tuberculosis, etc. Reasons for this optimism included low prices (Table 3) making goods generally affordable, minimal taxes and the potential for those aspiring to middle class or higher status to make money (Table 4). It was a country with widespread prosperity, at least as perceived by those who were established and economically well off.

Technological developments such as powered flight,[1] the automobile,[2] electricity, telephone, telegraph, typewriter, sewing machine, the Kodak Brownie camera, etc., all pointed to the role that technology would play in the future. These developments were viewed as examples of American ingenuity, which represented progress and fueled the perceived optimism of the times.

By 1900, the United States was one of the, if not the, richest countries on earth; yet it spite of this increasing wealth in terms of

Table 3.   Some Estimates of Selected Consumer Prices (1900–2000). Adapted From Various Sources: Britten and Mathless, 1998; The Economist: Dec. 21st, 2000; Time Magazine: April 13, 1998; http://www.albertsons.com (Figures Not Adjusted for Inflation).

	1900	2000
Dairy Products and Produce		
Eggs (dozen)	14¢	$1.12
Butter (lb.)	24¢	$2.35
Oranges (dozen)	20¢	$3.87
Lemons (dozen)	15¢	$3.98
Canned goods		
Golden cream corn	10¢	80¢
Boston baked beans	10¢	$1.99
Tomatoes	20¢	99¢
Sliced Peaches	25¢	$1.09
Staple Goods		
Sugar (lb)	4¢	43¢
Coffee (lb)	15¢	$5.99
Salt (lb)	0.2¢	$3.36
Automobiles Sold	4000	54 million

Table 4.   Some Demographic Estimates for the United States (1900–2000). Adapted From Various Sources: Britten and Mathless, 1998; The Economist: Dec. 21st, 2000; Time Magazine: April 13, 1998.

	1900	2000
Average life expectancy (years)	47.3	76.1
Birth rate per 1000	32.3	14.8
Death rate per 1000	17.2	4.9
Death rate per 1000 (under 1yr)	162.4	7.7
Population of the USA	76 million	249 million
Urban (%)	~30.4 million (40%)	~186.5 million (75%)
Rural (%)	~45.6 million (60%)	~62.2 million (25%)
Illiteracy rate %	10.7	~0.6
Total work force (%)	29.3 million (38%)	125 million (50%)
Average wage per hour	22¢	$11.82
Work hours per week	52	37.9
Average weekly income	$9.70	$435

GNP, the human costs were considerable. Fueling this new engine of progress were the immigrants from Europe. While the New World giant beckoned as the land of golden opportunities, the journey for the new immigrants was far from easy, involving untold hardships especially for those who were relatively poor.

An immigrant had to overcome many obstacles such as transit visas across European borders, identity cards, medical certificates, official documents verifying that taxes had been paid, military obligations completed, etc., as well as long waits at ports of embarkation.[8] By 1900 the cost of steerage had fallen enough so that individuals in relatively modest circumstances could afford the price of a ticket.[3,4]

The overwhelming majority of immigrants flocked to the larger cities increasing the populations of New York, Chicago and Philadelphia to over a million each by 1900. These newcomers, most of them poor, ended up working in the steel mills located in St. Louis, Pittsburgh, etc., or the mining towns of Pennsylvania or in the sweatshops of New York and Chicago.

The sights and sounds of this strange new country bewildered those who successfully entered the United States. Most immigrants searched out their country compatriots. This led to neighborhoods with familiar languages and foods, which had been settled earlier by fellow expatriates. The ethnic neighborhoods into which they settled tended to be composed of a few rundown streets with overcrowded tenants, open-air markets, and the numerous sweatshops. The lot of these poverty-stricken immigrants was one of living in disease-ridden slum tenements, with whole families crowded into single rooms in which all the activities of cooking, eating, sleeping were carried out. With little government assistance, immigrants were forced to rely upon each other. This bonding led to religious brotherhoods, community welfare associations, burial societies, labor unions, local political clubs, etc.[4]

Work available for the newcomers, largely single males, was hard, poorly paid and often dangerous. Those that had come from Eastern Europe and had some resources, tried to obtain employment doing what they did in the countries from which they had emigrated. They set up small businesses and shops. Those less fortunate ended up working for years at low wages[9] in the garment industry of New York at what became the numerous sweatshops.[10] They usually worked 12-hour days, six days a week.

Politically and otherwise naïve, especially in the workings of the American society, immigrants were often taken advantage of by ruthless and corrupt political bosses who were intent on lining their own pockets at the expense of those immigrants. Prejudice and bigotry were widespread. Disillusioned by the widespread pattern of prejudice, many immigrants gave up and returned to their homelands. In 1908, 395,000 left the U.S. and returned to their former countries.

Most immigrants, even if they managed to become proficient in English, spoke it with an accent. It was only the second generation that began to be accepted into the American mainstream, in part because of school system attendance, adoption of American customs and speaking English without a trace of an accent. This led to a gap between the generations. While many immigrants were able to leave the urban slums and enter the mainstream of American society, others were left behind, ending their lives and dreams without ever obtaining, even in a modest sense, the golden opportunities that drew them to the U.S. in the first place.

It was just such an immigrant, Isadore Sarnatzky, Bernie's father, who left his hometown in Belarus, Russia to migrate to the United States in 1907 in search for a better life for himself and his family. We take up his story in the next chapter.

Chapter 10

ROOTS IN BELARUS

Although Bernie's family ancestry has been traced to the early years of the 19th century, little of the family history is known until sometime in the middle of the 19th century.

Much of the following material was drawn from genealogical researches of family members Bernice Robin and Alice Sarnat who prepared the material for private family distribution. The total genealogical tree of the Sarnat clan consists of over 768 individuals over six generations from 1801 to the 1990's. While this number includes all marriages, live-in partners, and offspring up to that time, it is now understandably incomplete with respect to continuing births, marriages and deaths. Of those Sarnat family members that remained in Poland and Russia and who, unfortunately, found themselves in the way of Hitler's invading armies, at least 58 were lost to the Holocaust. This was 14.5% of the family members in the three generations at risk.

Bernie's paternal[1] great-grandparents were Nahum Sarnatzky[2] (1810–1875) and Yente Liebe who lived in the Tsarist Russian town of Skidel in the Belarussian (Belarus) part of the former USSR (Fig. 4; Family Tree). The nearest large city is Grodno (Hrodna), while Bialystok is the nearest town in modern Poland. The town of Skidel is positioned about 31 km directly east on the Grodno-Lida road. Today there are no Jewish families remaining in Skidel, although at one time it was a bustling Jewish commercial center specializing in leather tanning. Prior to the break-up of the

Soviet Union, Skidel was a regional headquarters of the Communist Party. This region was at the northwestern end of the Pale.[3,4] Skidel was one of the many small villages[5] that, in many ways, were typical for this region of Eastern Europe (Fig. 4).

Nahum and Yente had four children, three boys and one girl. They seem to have specialized in leather tanning and one of their boys (Avrom Sarnatzky, d. 1843) ran a leather factory in Skidel. Another boy, Mayer Sarnatzky (1843–1891), was Bernie's grandfather on his father's side. Mayer Sarnatzky and Gittle[6] Harawitz (1841–1925) married in 1859 and settled down in Skidel.

Skidel at the time of Bernie's grandfather (Mayer Sarnatzky) was a village of perhaps 1000 souls (Fig. 5), predominately Jewish.[7] The effects of the Holocaust and the march of armies, both German and Russian during World War II had taken their toll of the population. Mayer owned a general goods store in the town making him reasonably well off, certainly better off than many of the other village inhabitants. Nevertheless, life in such a village often consisted of a daily struggle for survival.

According to a widely held tale, one could gage the economic status of a family in the orthodox *shtetl* society of the Pale by their sugar usage, sugar being an expensive commodity at the time. Those who were relatively poor would hang a lump of sugar from the ceiling and as they drank their beverage such as tea, they would take a lick from this lump of sugar. Those who were somewhat better off would *dip* the lump into the tea in such a way that it would last for several cups. Those who were affluent would place a lump of sugar *into* the tea. Finally, the very prosperous would use granulated sugar and would put one or two teaspoons into the tea.

The next chapter outlines the paths taken by Bernie's family members as they left the Old World and began a new life with their migration to the New World.

Chapter 11

EMIGRATION TO CHICAGO

Mayer Sarnatzky and his wife Gittle had nine surviving children out of eleven, six girls and three boys. The next to last were fraternal twins (b. 1875) and the last were triplets, born in 1878. Of the triplets, Isadore (Bernie's father) was the only one to survive. His birth weight must have been somewhere between two and four pounds. Since incubators were unknown at the time, what his post-natal care consisted of is anyone's guess. Presumably, he was kept close to the breast for warmth and food; nevertheless, it is amazing that he did survive. Survive he did indeed, living to the age of 84. We shall pick up his story again subsequently.

The oldest of the six surviving female siblings was called Chamke or Malka Sarnatzky who eventually married a non-Jewish Russian officer. This resulted, according to Orthodox tradition, in her being permanently disowned by the rest of the Sarnatzky family. Her descendants are unknown. It is speculated that this marriage with the Russian officer may have acted to reduce the local marriage chances for the remaining women, which in turn may also have acted as one of the many catalysts influencing emigration to the United States.

Another female sibling who did not immigrate until the early 1900's was Dobbe Liebe Sarnatzky (1865–1945) who married Alexander Ziskin Kagen (1857–1932). Her husband was an unusually talented man who was honored by the Tzar for having helped organize the first census of Russia. He was a gymnasium (high school) graduate who had a liquor license, which was considered unusual for a Jew,[1] and was fluent in ten languages.

The other four female siblings, all eventually migrated to Chicago, although one (Eshka Sarnatzky, see below) eventually returned to Europe. The first of the four siblings who chose to emigrate was Rose Sarnatzky (1869–1948), who moved to Chicago sometime before 1892. It is presumed that she knew someone there. The second one, Eshka Sarnatzky (1870–1941?) who had traveled to the U.S. for the 1893 Chicago World's Fair, stayed for a year with Rose but returned to Skidel to marry her much loved boyfriend. Unfortunately, she later moved to Warsaw against the family's advice.[1] She probably died in 1941 at the Grodno concentration camp. All her family members died in the Holocaust as well, with the exception of one child (Anne Kane) who escaped in 1943 via France and Portugal and arrived at Baltimore on the S.S. Serpa Pinto which was named after a Portuguese explorer of South Africa and colonial administrator (1846–1900). This was the last ship to have landing rights in the U.S. during the war.

The third sibling was Boshke (later Bessie) Sarnatzky (1868–1938) who immigrated first to New Jersey and then to Chicago in 1907. The fourth sibling was Zlotke Sarnatzky, one of the twins born in 1875, who arrived circa 1924. Finally, the other twin, was Nahum Zelig Sarnatzky, who died in Mexico City.

Of the other surviving male siblings, Israel Sarnatzky (1869–1917), Bernie's uncle, migrated to the U.S. in 1908. His reasons for doing so are not clear since he was well established in Skidel. He owned a leather and footwear factory, which with 44 employees in 1900 was the largest factory in Skidel. Israel died in 1917 in New York of a ruptured appendix. He became ill on the Sabbath and the family would not take him to the hospital.[1] Bernie, five years old in 1917, remembers a period of mourning when the mirrors in the house were covered and then in the evening several men in black came over to the house to pray. He knew this had something to do with his uncle who had died in New York.

Migration from Russia of Isadore Sarnatzky

Bernie's father, Isadore Sarnatzky[2] (1878–1964), was the last of the nine surviving siblings born to Mayer and Gittle Sarnatzky. When Isadore was born, he was one of a set of triplets, as mentioned earlier, and the only survivor as the other two died at birth. Given the primitive state of pre- and post-natal care in such a predominantly Jewish Russian village or *shtetl*, this would not be altogether unexpected. Mortality rates were quite high, especially with multiple births.

In 1901, at the age of 23, Isadore married a girl named Fanny (born in 1880), from a nearby town of Volkovysk about 56 km south of Skidel and also 92 km directly east of Bialystok (Fig. 4). This was probably a typically arranged marriage in which the bridal party traveled by horse and wagon over dirt roads. In a typical Jewish fashion, the wedding celebration was said to have lasted about a week. In spite of relatively little formal education, his new wife was not only quite intelligent, being fluent in languages such as German, Russian, Polish and Yiddish, but also a 'take charge' person in that she quickly adjusted to Isadore's family life by helping run the general store. This general store had been in the family for a while, being owned by Isadore's parents.

In 1902, they had their first child named Jacob. About sixteen months later in 1903, they had a second child, this time a girl named Tena. It was around this time that Isadore contemplated the possibility of leaving Skidel. Conditions in the Pale had deteriorated. The ever-present threat of pogroms as well as potential conscription into the Russian army for a period of 25 years, also unattractive, acted as a catalyst for emigration. In addition, a strong inducement was the possibility of good employment in the United States.

In 1907 Isadore left Skidel for the United States. He arrived via the S.S. Merion and entered through Ellis Island. When Isadore arrived in the U.S., he briefly visited his sister Boshke who was then living in New Jersey but would eventually move to Chicago. In Chicago, Isadore had a job waiting for him working for his sister.

Rose's spouse, Hyman Schultz, who owned a retail store[3] at the time, dealing in sundries in the commercial district just west of downtown Chicago. He was ostensibly looking for a sales clerk to help him. Soon after his arrival, Isadore became the principal clerk responsible for selling candy, cigars, cigarettes, snuff, pipes, knives and other sundries. Once employed, he worked long hours, began to learn English, adopt American customs and settle down. Chicago became Isadore's permanent home. He eventually ran the whole store. Toward the end of the first decade (1909), he was able to bring his wife, Fanny, and their two young children, Jacob and Tena, to Chicago (Fig. 8).

Settling Down in Chicago

What kind of a man was Isadore Sarnatzky? Bernie's earliest recollections of his father begin around the age of four (1916). As his father worked long hours, Bernie rarely saw him for any length of time during the workweek including half-days on Saturdays. The only exception was on Sundays when the family would go on outings.

When Bernie arose around 8 in the morning, his father had already left for work. His father usually returned around 7 or 8 in the evening after the rest of the family had eaten their suppers so that he would have to dine late.

Bernie's recollections paint a picture of a man who was generous and caring, who rarely raised his voice at home to chastise his children. Bernie recalled that he was always well groomed and very neat in appearance. However, his intellectual abilities were not exceptional and even his business acumen was not particularly noteworthy. His strengths lay in other directions such as his ability to relate to others in a very personal way, as exemplified by the following story.

When Bernie was in college (1929) and working part-time in his father's drugstore,[4,5] he recalled that during the twenty years that his father owned that drugstore at 57th Street and Blackstone (discussed more fully in Chapter 12) just off the University of

Chicago campus, that his father really enjoyed running the drug-store, especially serving the people who came in. He evidently got extreme pleasure out of helping others. As an example, Bernie related how many college students living nearby would come in and having run out of their allowance, were allowed to charge items such as a five-cent coke or a fifteen-cent sandwich, and he would often forget to keep track of the charges. At the end of the month, a statement of those charges would be itemized and sent to the student for collection. Collecting the money owed was not always easy and the drugstore lost money running these charge accounts.

During the Depression, to make ends meet, Bernie pleaded with his father to eliminate these charge accounts but his father would not consider it, and so the drugstore continued to lose money with the charge accounts. Nevertheless, Isadore was always helping, giving in extra ways and catering to their needs. Small wonder then that everyone who came in contact with him loved him. Although a foreigner who spoke with an accent, Isadore was accommodating, friendly and well liked by the faculty, staff and stu-dents at the University of Chicago who frequented the drugstore. It was his presence that made the drugstore greatly appreciated not only as a family enterprise but also as an institution fondly remem-bered by those who lived in the neighborhood.

As the drugstore was generally busy, people had the impres-sion that Bernie's father was earning a good living, when in real-ity the family was just getting by. Nevertheless, as owner of the drugstore, Isadore's life revolved around it as he opened it up at 8:00 in the morning and closed it at midnight, seven days a week.

While Bernie did not have any idea as to the exact family worth, the family always lived modestly, so that although they, as others, had to struggle during the depression of the 1930's, they did not have to deal with some of the more severe financial hardships that beset so many others. Bernie's father felt that money was there to be spent and never begrudged the demands of the family given that they were reasonable.

Bernie recalled that when his sister was 12 (circa 1916) his father liked to indulge her so he bought her a muff and feather boa (Fig. 8). He must have spent 10 or 12 dollars, a fair sum at that time (probably a good part of a week's salary). Upon arriving at home with the gifts, Bernie's mother was appalled and said that he should not have wasted the money. Thus, one could say that Bernie's mother was the thrifty one while his father was not, a pattern characteristic for most of their lives.

In 1920, Bernie's parents had now saved enough money to buy a building composed of three apartments at 3236 Evergreen Avenue located on the other side of Humboldt Park but still on the Northwest side of Chicago. This was then what could be considered as an upwardly mobile Jewish neighborhood. The Sarnats were now well underway and climbing the economic ladder. That year they moved into the second floor of the three-storey apartment building and now being landlords, rented out floors one and three. The former owner (he was now paying rent) by the name of Diamond continued to live on the first floor, but moved out within several months. The tenant on the third floor was called Richardson who worked for the Texaco oil company.

When Bernie was around nine (1921), his father came down with pneumonia. During his father's illness, Bernie recalled that a series of heated glass cups were placed on the skin creating suction that, in some old medical way, was intended to heal. His father nearly died. Luckily, the family did call in a specialist who then had him hospitalized. The doctor indicated that it was a matter of life or death and that it would be resolved one way or another in the next eight days. Bernie's father did go through a crisis; there was lobar pneumonia (fluid in the lungs) but he recovered. Had Bernie's father died at that time, the future of the family might have turned out very differently.

Another incident that Bernie recalled concerned his father's brother-in-law. Hyman Schultz owned a summer home in Western Michigan at Paw Paw Lake. His brother-in-law would go up there for the summer for two or three months leaving Bernie's father in charge of the retail store. Eventually in 1932, Bernie's parents, largely because of the frugality of Bernie's mother, saved enough money to allow them to also begin building a modest summer home about a block away from his brother-in-law. They were to spend many enjoyable summers there. It was there that Bernie's father loved to spend his summers, when he could get away from the cares of work. In fact, in the year of 1934, he took the whole summer off, leaving Bernie in sole charge at the drugstore. Bernie was only 22 at the time. It was also while vacationing at the summer home that, in 1951, Bernie's mother died quite suddenly from a coronary.

The next chapter takes a closer look at how Bernie's life revolved around his father's drugstore experiences.

BACKGROUND AND THE SARNAT FAMILY (1912–1997)

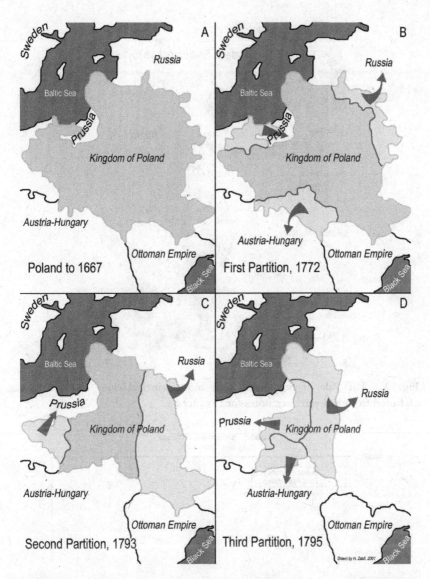

Fig. 1. The three Partitions of Poland (1772–1795). Arrows depict land acquisitions by the respective adjacent countries (see Chapter 2).

Notes: Open circles — city forbidden to Jewish settlement. Only Riga was forbidden to *new* Jewish settlement after 1835. Stippled sections — the one on the eastern border refers to provinces where Jewish settlement in villages was forbidden. The one on the western border refers to the region forbidden to *new* Jewish settlement (see Chapter 3).

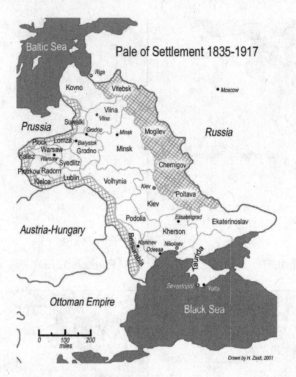

Fig. 2. The Pale of Settlement with some principal cities and provinces. (Adapted from Ettinger[3]; see notes for Chapter 3).

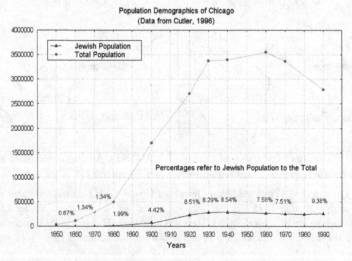

Fig. 3. Population of Chicago (1850–1990) (see Chapter 8).

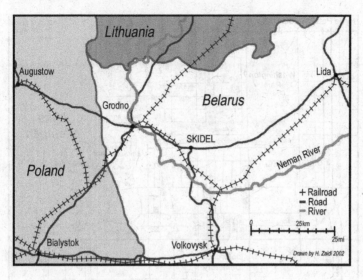

Fig. 4. Location of Skidel, Belarus (see Chapter 10).

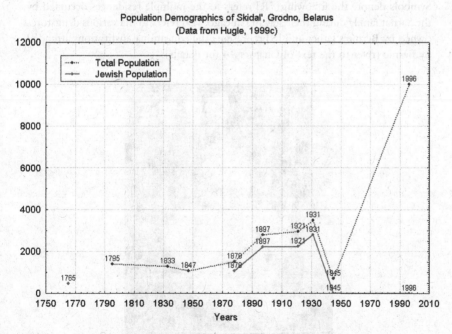

Fig. 5. Population of Skidel (1765–1996) (see Chapter 10).

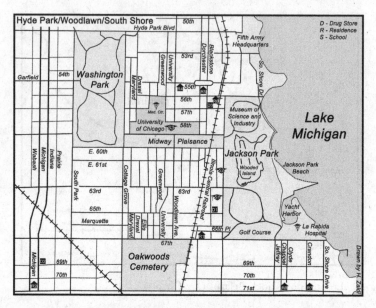

Fig. 6. Map of the Hyde Park–Woodlawn–South Shore regions of Chicago. Symbols denote the following: [R] refers to the multiple residences occupied by the Sarnat family during their stay in Chicago, [D] refers to the various drugstores owned by Bernie's father and [S] represents the educational institutions attended by Bernie (refer to the text of Chapter 14 for details).

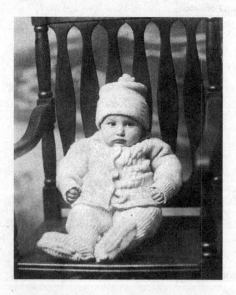

Fig. 7. Infant Bernie, Chicago.

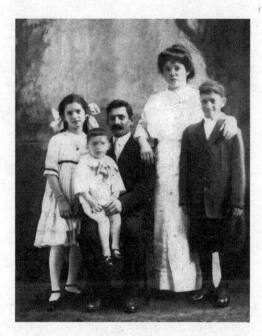

Fig. 8.   1916. The Sarnat Family: Tena, Bernie, Isadore, Fanny, Jack.

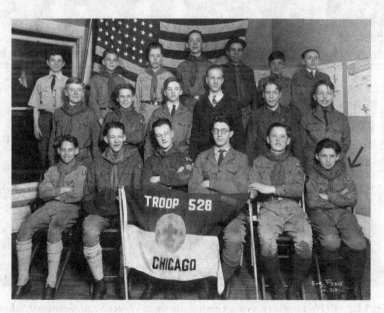

Fig. 9.   1925. Bernie (*arrow*), Boy Scout Troop 528. Church of the Redeemer, 66th Place and Blackstone Avenue, Chicago.

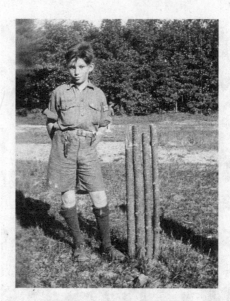

Fig. 10.   1926. Bernie, Boy Scout Summer Camp at Owassippe, Muskeogen, Michigan.

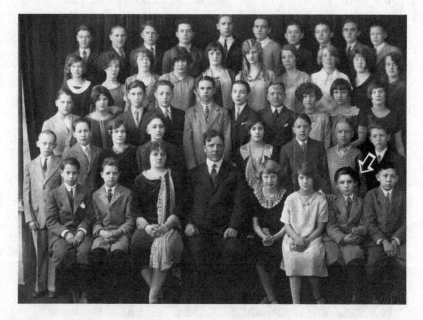

Fig. 11.   1926. Bernie (*arrow*), Graduation from Walter Scott Grammar School, 64th and Blackstone Avenue, Chicago.

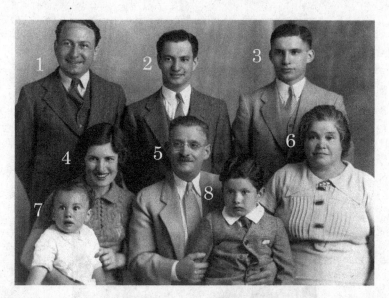

Fig. 12. 1936. Bernie's graduation from the University of Chicago, Medical School, 1936; Received MD degree, 1937. 1, Leo Spira; 2, Jack; 3, Bernie; 4, Tena Sarnat Spira; 5, Isadore; 6, Fanny; 7, Richard Spira; 8, Robert Spira.

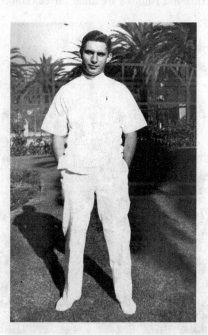

Fig. 13. 1936. Bernie. Internship, Los Angeles County Hospital, November.

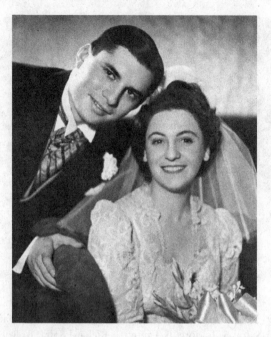

Fig. 14.   1941. Bernie and Rhoda's wedding on December 25th, Windermere East Hotel, Chicago.

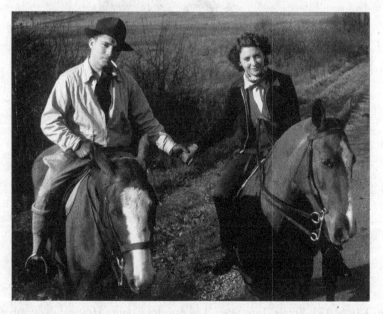

Fig. 15.   1942. Bernie and Rhoda on their honeymoon in Biloxi, Mississippi.

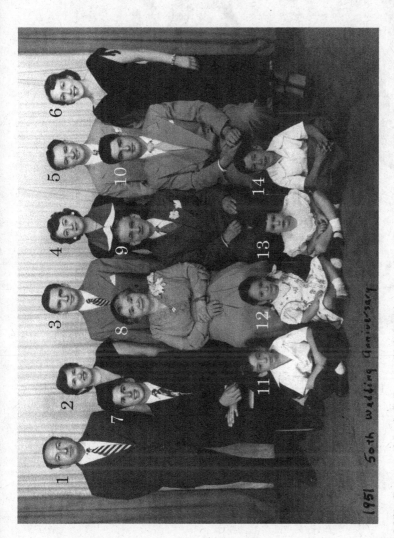

Fig. 16. 1951. Fanny and Isadore Sarnat 50th Golden Wedding Anniversary Family at Large Dinner at the Shoreland Hotel, Chicago. 1, Leo Spira; 2, Tena Sarnat Spira; 3, Bernie; 4, Rhoda; 5, Jack; 6, Edna Siegel Sarnat; 7, Richard Spira; 8, Fanny; 9, Isadore; 10, Robert Spira; 11, Gerard Sarnat; 12, Joan Sarnat; 13, Susan Sarnat; 14, William Sarnat.

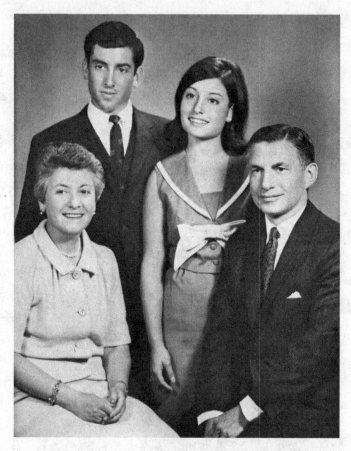

Fig. 17.   1965. Rhoda, Gerry, Joan, Bernie. 616 N. Maple Drive, Beverly Hills, California.

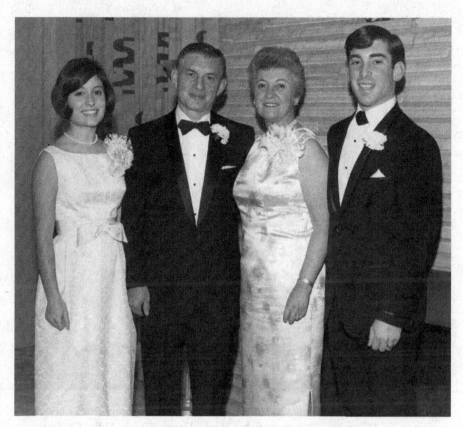

Fig. 18.   1966. Joan, Bernie, Rhoda, Gerry. The four Sarnats at Rhoda and Bernies 25th Wedding Anniversary sit down dinner on December 28th for some 65 family and friends at 616 N. Maple Drive, Beverly Hills, California.

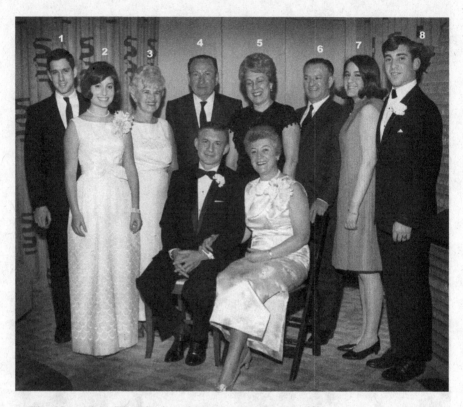

Fig. 19.   1966. The Rhoda and Bernie Sarnat 25th wedding anniversary sit down dinner on December 28th at 616 N. Maple Drive, Beverly Hills, California, December 28th. 1, William Sarnat; 2, Joan; 3, Tena Sarnat Spira; 4, Leo Spira; 5, Edna Sarnat; 6, Jack; 7, Susan Sarnat; 8, Gerry. Missing, Robert and Richard Spira.

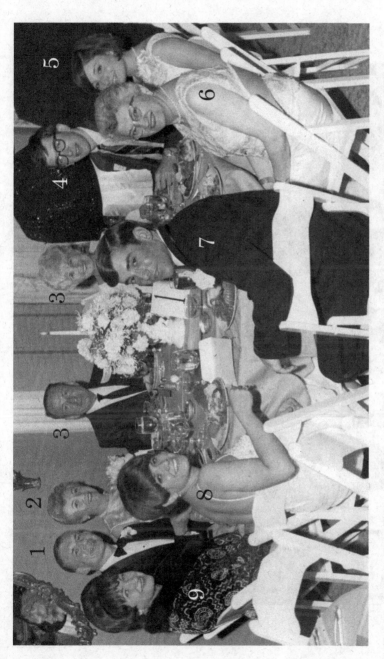

Fig. 20. 1966. The Rhoda and Bernie Sarnat's 25th Wedding Anniversary Cocktail and Sit Down Dinner Party on December 28th at their home at 616 N. Maple Drive, Beverly Hills, California. HOST TABLE. 1, Bernie; 2, Rhoda; 3, Leo Spira (Master of Ceremonies); 3, Tena Spira; 4, Jon Greenwald (Joan's Date); 5, Joan; 6, Esther Schour; 7, Gerry; 8, Barbara Goodhill (Gerry's Date); 9, Estey Graham. There were 65 guests, relatives and friends at seven tables.

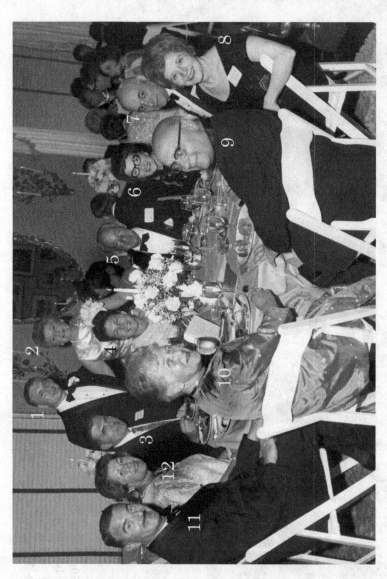

Fig. 21. 1966. Rhoda and Bernie Sarnat 25th Wedding Anniversary Cocktail and Sit Down Dinner on December 28th at their home at 616 N. Maple Drive, Beverly Hills, California, December 28. 1, Bernie; 2, Rhoda; 3, Irving Janis; 4, Marjorie Graham Janis; 5, Victor Graham; 6, Olga Graham; 7, Ralph Colton; 8, Elsie Gerard Colton (Rhoda's sister); 9, Ralph Gerard (Rhoda's brother); 10, Frosty Gerard; 11, Manny Fineman; 12, Evelyn Fineman.

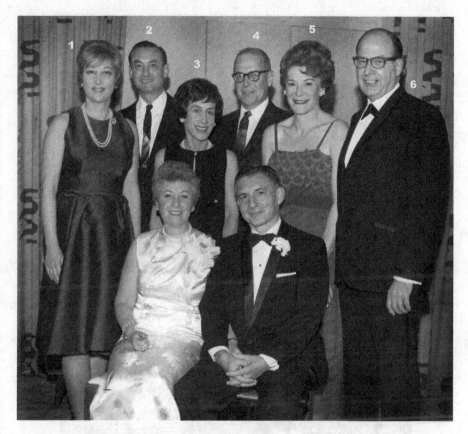

Fig. 22.   1966. The Hungry Four (now Eight). 1, Carol Colby; 2, Bernie Colby; 3, Peggy Kreisman; 4, Herbert Kreisman; 5, Dorothy Shanedling; 6, Philip Shanedling. Bernie and Rhoda's 25th Wedding Anniversary on December 28th.

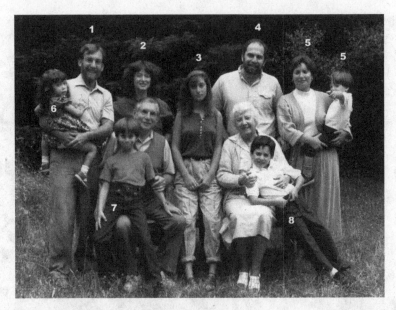

Fig. 23. 1987. The Bernie and Rhoda Sarnat Family at Mendocino, California. 1, Gerry with Emma, 6; 2, Lela; 3, Zoe; 4, David Hoffman; 5, Joan Sarnat Hoffman; 5, Michael Hoffman; 7, Eli Sarnat; 8, Jascha Hoffman.

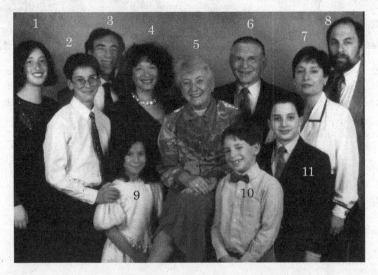

Fig. 24. 1991. The Bernie and Rhoda Sarnat Family. 50th Wedding Anniversary on a Mexican Cruise. 1, Zoe Sarnat; 2, Eli Sarnat; 3, Gerry; 4, Lela Sarnat; 5, Rhoda; 6, Bernie; 7, Joan Sarnat Hoffman; 8, David Hoffman; 9, Emma Sarnat; 10, Michael Hoffman; 11, Jascha Hoffman.

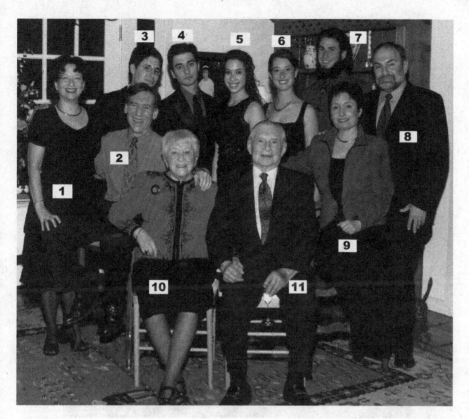

Fig. 25. 1997. The Bernie and Rhoda Sarnat Family. Bernie's 85th Birthday Celebration at Gerry and Lela's home in Portola Valley, California. 1, Lela; 2, Gerry; 3, Michael Hoffman; 4, Jascha Hoffman; 5, Emma Sarnat; 6, Zoe Sarnat; 7, Eli Sarnat; 8, David Hoffman; 9, Joan Sarnat Hoffman; 10, Rhoda; 11, Bernie.

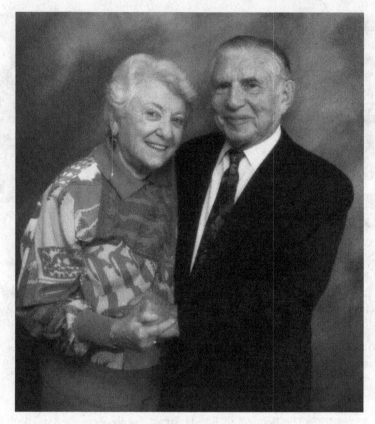

Fig. 26.   1997. Bernie and Rhoda.

Chapter 12

RETAIL STORE TO DRUGSTORES

In the 1920's, numerous relatives of Bernie's father were pharmacists and owned drugstores in the Chicago area. Such drugstores were extremely common; one could find them virtually on every city block. They were often family run and prided themselves on personal service. At one time, there were ten or more of these drugstores owned by nephews and cousins as well as one wholesale drug company, General Drug Co., owned by Sam Sarnatzky, within the expanding Sarnat lineage. In addition, Bernie's brother, Jack, was working in one of the family drugstores by this time. These factors eventually provided the catalyst for Isadore to also consider the possibility of owning a drugstore.

Bernie's father had now accumulated enough money to buy out his brother-law, Hyman Schultz. So in 1921, with the help of a partner named Friedman, Isadore bought his brother-in-law's general store dealing in tobacco and sundries, allowing his brother-in-law to retire in his fifties. After about nine months to a year, the partner wanted to withdraw and Isadore bought him out as well. However, by 1922, he found that running the retail store alone did not prove to be satisfactory either, so he decided to sell the store.

With the proceeds, and having little to do, he began to look around for another business venture. Consequently, in 1923 Isadore had the necessary funds for the purchase of a drugstore located at 65th and Blackstone Avenue on the Southside of Chicago.

Although not a full pharmacist, Bernie's older brother, Jack, now twenty-one, had become an assistant pharmacist in one of the numerous drugstores owned by the extended Sarnat family, started work in Isadore's drugstore. Since the drugstore was located on the Southside and they lived on the Northwest side of Chicago, this entailed a one-hour trip on the elevated train (the "el") each way. As the drugstore was open from eight in the morning until midnight, this made for long and arduous days for Isadore and Jack who at that time was a second-year dental student. Bernie fondly recalled being awakened up after midnight to partake of some ice cream brought from the drugstore. This rather arduous trip continued for some months until the family moved to the Southside when Bernie then transferred to Walter Scott elementary school at 64th and Blackstone Avenue in September 1923.

Isadore thus ran his first drugstore venture with the help of Jack and a full-time pharmacist for three years (Bernie started here as delivery boy) and had built it up so that it was doing quite well. At the end of three years, Isadore found out that the landlord would not renew the drugstore lease. In fact, three months before the lease had expired he found out that the owner had leased the property to someone else some months previously. This led to a traumatic period and Isadore had to look for a new location.

He found an empty store in 1926, several blocks south and two miles west of the first drugstore. This building, located at 69th and Indiana Avenue had been a drugstore at one time. This was a Scandinavian neighborhood and it took Isadore some time to get re-established. He started building up the business in the second drugstore until, within two or three years, it was doing nicely.

In 1928, the clerk who had been working for Isadore insisted on buying the drugstore and Isadore agreed. The clerk had done a wonderful job in developing and expanding the drugstore over the ensuing years. During this time, Bernie continued to work as a delivery boy, swept and mopped the floor, took out the trash and shelved stock for this clerk after he had bought the drugstore.

After Isadore had sold this second drugstore to his clerk, he worked for a time for one of his nephews in his drugstore located at Marquette Road (66th St.) and Kenwood. This drugstore was just 2½ blocks away from the one Isadore had owned previously. Eventually Bernie also left the employ of the clerk who had bought Isadore's second drugstore and went to work for a cousin of his in another drugstore. The Sarnat family had now moved to Yates Avenue in South Shore.

Isadore bought his third and last drugstore in May of 1929, which was located at 1438 East 57th Street, actually 57th Street and Blackstone Avenue, just off the campus of the University of Chicago. This drugstore was located in Hyde Park, a prestigious area at that time, solidly middle and upper-middle class. This was a drugstore he liked very much

Bernie's father suffered two big financial blows. He had bought the drugstore, near the University of Chicago, but did not realize that the University was not in session during the months of August/September, so business plummeted during that time. Then in October came the stock market crash. Times became quite difficult, but the family struggled and survived. Bernie, who was now a student at the University of Chicago, offered to drop out and help by clerking full-time in the drugstore. His offer, however, was refused in no uncertain terms and his parents found the necessary money for tuition.

This third drugstore was initially rather run down because the previous owner was more interested in running after women than running the drugstore. Therefore, this became a wonderful opportunity for Isadore to build up the store business. Although within a two-block area there were three drugstores, there was enough business to allow all three to prosper.

The drugstore had a soda fountain and served light luncheon sandwiches at 15 and 20 cents each. Malted milks were 20 cents, a coca cola was 5 cents, ice cream sundaes and sodas were 15 cents, and soup was also available. Candy was sold in bulk and boxes. A pound of Whitman's sampler, a well-known and exclusive type of candy, was $1.50 a box. The Whitman salesman was excellent and returned periodically to see that they were well stocked. After Christmas he came by to change the markings on each box to reflect Valentine's Day. After that he would change the markings for Easter, for Mother's Day and so on throughout the year. Also sold were toiletries such as perfumes, lipsticks and cosmetics as well as cigarettes, tobacco, cigars and snuff. A carton of cigarettes (10 packs) went for 99 cents. Also sold were beer, fine wines and whiskey as well as newspapers and magazines, and yes, even pharmaceuticals and prescriptions.

At that time prescriptions were compounded. A physician would prescribe several drugs and these would be triturated (mixed) using a mortar and pestle and made into capsules or powders. Although some items were dispensed as pills, that procedure was not nearly as common as today.

In addition, there was a rental library. It was first run by Marian Books and subsequently Beverly Books took it over. Bernie discovered that they were padding the profits by some 30% so this part of the business was turned over to Tena, Bernie's older sister, for management. It was renamed Bob's Book Shelf, after her older son, and books were rented out at the rate of 10 cents for the first three days and 2 cents for every day thereafter. At this time the Chicago Tribune sold at 2 cents a copy.

Part of the neighborliness of their drug store at 57th and Blackstone Avenue was displayed at every Thanksgiving and Christmas. A week or two before these holidays Bernie's father would hold a raffle. Previous to that time, he would have issued a double ticket for every purchase. One of the tickets would be deposited into a large bowl, the customer would retain the other ticket, and then, at a prearranged date, usually seven o'clock in the evening, the drawing would be held. Two or three turkeys, boxes of candy, cosmetics and other desirable merchandise would be in the raffle. It was a very popular event. The entire store would be jammed with people with some of them overflowing to the outside. As a result, a microphone was required to call out each number after one of the customers had picked a ticket out of the bowl. There was always a great deal of interest and enthusiasm generated by the customers. It would always be a highly successful event, and was continued for several years.

Another popular item was "sprinkles." These were 1 mm by 6 mm chocolate bits. An ice cream cone (5 cents) was dipped into these bits and would come out chocolate covered. In the 1930s, this became quite the rage off-campus and many people came from far and near for this popular item. When Bernie's son was at Harvard in 1963, he also became acquainted with this fashion known then as "jimmies."

Two blocks away, for a distance of about a mile, on 55th street, between Dorchester and Cottage Grove, there was a drugstore on just about every corner. At 55th and Dorchester there was a Walgreen's drugstore, one of the very early ones, long before Walgreen's became a national chain. However, with the increasing use of automobiles providing greater mobility, these mom and pop drugstores began to disappear and in their place, there appeared the regional chains of self-service drugstores.

Drugstore Clientele

Isadore Sarnat was beloved by both the drugstore staff and his customers and for very good reasons. He was most accommodating and understanding. For example, numerous University of Chicago co-eds would not hesitate to discuss their personal problems or being short of cash with him. He would often allow them to charge items with little hope of payment. If customers wanted something that the drugstore did not carry, he would go out of his way to try to acquire it for them.

Patrons of the Sarnat Drug Company as it was then called included frequent, regular, as well some irregular visits by prominent members of the University of Chicago (U of C) faculty as well as other neighbors. Some of the individuals included the famous and not so famous such as: Alf Alvin, University of Chicago (U of C) nephrologist; Dinsmore, Superintendent of Billings Hospital; Kornhauser, University of Chicago psychologist; Morris Fishbein, Editor of the Journal of the American Medical Association; Ralph Gerard, Neurophysiologist, U of C; Esmond Long, Pulmonologist, U of C; Thomas Park, geneticist, U of C;

Sidney Portis, gastroenterologist, private practice and Rush medical College; Rukeyser (father and son), security analysts; Scammon, anatomist and MD, U of C; Dallas Phemister, Professor and Head of the Department of Surgery, U of C; Solomon and Carl Strouse (father and son), internists and on the staff of Rush Medical College; Helen Wright, Dean, School of Social Work, U of C; Swenson, psychologist, U of C; Clifton and Garrick Utley (father and son), News and political commentary; Franck, physicist, U of C; Stanton Friedberg (father and son), both Department Heads at Rush medical college; Robert Maynard Hutchins (President of U of C); etc.

Bernie recalled others, for example, Paul Douglas, a professor of economics at the U of C, who later became Alderman of the fifth ward and then U.S. Senator Douglas, a Democrat, would wait in the evening outside the drugstore for the truck that dropped off the Chicago Tribune. He wanted to see what the Tribune had to say. Douglas would take the bundle of papers into the drugstore and put them on the counter. He would then take one paper over to the soda fountain and sit there reading it from front page to the back page. When he was finished, he would fold it up and put it back. He would never buy the paper, as that would be patronizing the Chicago Tribune, a Republican paper.

Another recollection was that of Frank Banes who was warden of Virginia State Prison before the University of Chicago brought him in to be Chair of the Department of Public Policy. He and his wife would often come in to the drugstore to visit with Isadore. They were good friends and Isadore would be invited to their Christmas parties.

Another customer was Percival Bailey, a famous neurosurgeon who was Chairman of the Department of Neurosurgery at the U of C. He evidently had spent some time during his education in Paris and became quite devoted to French wines. He would have Bernie's father order a case of a specific French wine which he liked. Always accommodating, he was happy to do this for him. Later (1939) Bailey transferred to the University of Illinois on the Westside of Chicago and Bernie would frequently drive Bailey there as this was also where Bernie would go each day. At one time Bailey told Bernie that he considered him as "one of his boys" even though Bernie never became one of his residents.

Another recollection of Bernie's involved Douglas Waple, head of Library Science at the U of C, who would come in to the drugstore every Friday around 5pm to check out the latest detective fiction at the rental book library and purchase a bottle of whiskey. Bernie's father would always lay away for him the latest detective story that had come in. Dr. Waple would go home on Friday evenings and presumably settle down after dinner to read the detective story with a libation at his side.

Isadore's Retirement

In 1948, Isadore sold the drugstore to the wife of one of his clerks who, in turn, sold it to another one of Isadore's clerks. Throughout the next decade it retained the name of Sarnat Drug Company. The drugstore had been owned by Bernie's father from 1929 to 1948, and lasted another ten years or so under the same name but different management, until 1958 or 1959. With the changing neighborhood, the next generation of clerks eliminated the wine, liquor and beer, as well as the soda fountain, and practically limit the drugstore to just pharmaceuticals and prescriptions. As business dropped off considerably, the pharmacist owner retired, because by then the neighborhood around the University of Chicago was radically deteriorating. Eventually a typewriter store replaced the drugstore. Subsequently, the typewriter store also went out of business. In the last several decades, a Greek restaurant is on the site of where the Sarnat drugstore was once situated. Bernie has frequented this now popular restaurant, gazing down at the same tile floor that he used to mop as a youth in the wintertime, which brought back a flood of memories.

In 1949, Isadore finally retired, and he and his wife began to spend long summers in Western Michigan at Paw Paw Lake where they had owned a home since 1932. In June of 1951, a golden wedding anniversary party was held for the family at large. Also in

1951, with the sudden death of Bernie's mother at 71, in August of that year from a coronary, his father disposed of their apartment where they had lived since 1933 and he moved to South Shore, where Bernie and his two older siblings lived. He had a nicely furnished apartment there. In 1960 he moved in with Bernie's sister who lived nearby. After a few years it became apparent that he required more assistance than she could give him so he was moved into a nursing home about 1962 where he died in December of 1964 at the age of 86.

Chapter 13

ELEMENTARY LESSONS

Bernard George Sarnat was the third and last child of Isadore and Fanny Sarnatzky (Fig. 7 and Fig. 8) who had migrated from Russia a few years before. Bernie was born in Chicago on September 1, 1912 at Michael Reese Hospital located on the Southside at the lakefront. Bernie's two siblings at the time of his birth were Jacob aged ten and a sister named Tena aged eight. According to Rhoda, Bernie's spouse (to be introduced in her own right in Chapter 19), Bernie's mother, at first, did not plan on a third child and went to the Riverview amusement park on the suggestion of some of her lady friends, and rode the Bobs, a scary high ride in the hope of having a miscarriage. However, as luck would have it, she emerged with her fetus intact and once born, little Bernie became the family favorite, an earnest, serious little boy.

At birth, he was given the Hebrew name of Benyomen or Benjamin Gershen Sarnatzky after an uncle who had died. Living in a mixed neighborhood and sensitive to being immigrants, especially Jewish ones, family members tried to assimilate as rapidly as possible into the larger Chicago community in any way possible. This was a widespread pattern characteristic of many immigrant groups, not just Jews. Consequently, Bernie's older brother, who hated his name of Jacob, changed it to Jack. In the same vein, rather than Benyomen or Benjamin Gershen, an anglicized version was chosen for Bernie: Bernard George. When Isadore, their father, became a U.S. citizen in 1918, he also changed the family name from Sarnatzky to Sarnat. Within a couple of years, Bernie's birth certificate was also duly modified to reflect this name change.[1]

Prior to his fourth birthday (around 1915), Bernie and his family lived on a street known as Raymond Court on the Northwest side of Chicago, a more or less lower/middle class area. The family that lived upstairs was named Kotin. Esther Kotin, one of the daughters, was instrumental in bringing Bernie and his future wife Rhoda together in 1941, but more of this later (see Chapter 19). To help with expenses, boarders were taken in. By his fourth birthday, the family had moved to North Maplewood Avenue, generally in the same Northwest side of Chicago. This was a rented two-story building with the family living on the second floor and the owner, an attorney named Raff, living on the first floor. Bernie recalled it was stove heated with his mother bringing up buckets of coal to heat the apartment. Since Bernie's father left early and returned late from work at the retail store, he would only see him just before his bedtime and on Sundays. Bernie also recalled a man on a bicycle coming in the evenings to light the gas lamps on the street.

One of Bernie's earliest recollections occurred on September 1st, 1916. As he had just turned four, he was given a birthday party by his sister, Tena, and a cousin Celia. Celia eventually became the mother-in-law of William Rivkin, Ambassador to Luxembourg and Gambia, as well as grandmother of Jonathan Alter, Senior Editor Columnist for Newsweek. Among his birthday gifts were a little play fireman's hat, shield and axe. Toys with which Bernie happily played in the backyard where there was a cherry tree, which, in contrast to George Washington, he did not cut down. However, he did eat the cherries.

When Bernie was around four his mother attempted to send him off to kindergarten but being too young, he was promptly sent home. At this age, Bernie also recalled another memorable experience. He was taken for a horse and wagon ride by the milkman who made his rounds in the neighborhood.

Bernie eventually entered kindergarten at von Humboldt School where he also attended first grade. There in 1917, Bernie made friends with a boy, Alan Lieberman, a few doors down who became a playmate for several months until Bernie and his family moved again. Bernie lost contact with Alan until 1932 when as a sophomore at the University of Chicago he was approached by a student who asked him if he was Bernie Sarnat. Bernie then recognized Alan as his playmate of 1917. Bernie remained in contact with him. He became a prominent psychiatrist as Chief of Elgin State Hospital and eventually retired to Palm Springs, California, where he died in 2002.

When Bernie was six, sometime in 1918, he also recalled a time that was later called the "false armistice." Everyone was excited and there were boxes burning in the street that the Great War was finally over only to find out that the celebration had been premature.[2]

Another incident that Bernie, now aged six, remembered involved his father and his older brother. The three of them were at the store one Saturday morning and during a quiet time they sat Bernie on a high stool near a stove that kept the store warm, and proceeded to give him a haircut.

In 1918, Bernie's family again moved once more, this time to West Iowa Street. This was still located on the Northwest side of Chicago, but Bernie's family was starting to progress up the economic scale. This was a large three-story corner building in a predominantly Jewish neighborhood. It had steam heat instead of the coal stoves present at the former location on North Maplewood Avenue. Again, they lived on the second floor where they rented out one bedroom to a woman boarder to supplement their income. The third floor was rented out by the owner while the first floor contained a delicatessen. Behind the delicatessen, there was a small rear apartment.

In 1918, Bernie entered the second grade at Chopin Elementary School. While in the second grade at Chopin, Bernie recalled that he became the major player in a school play. The third grade was the last one that Bernie attended at Chopin as the family moved again.

When Bernie was seven years old his father had one week's vacation and took him via steamer from Navy Pier overnight to

Benton Harbor where they stayed at a resort. At that time in 1919, Benton Harbor was administered by the House of David Israelites. The men had beards and long hair and believed in polygamy. They had an amusement park, a baseball team and ran the trolley cars.

When Bernie was about eight he recalled coming home on a Saturday to find that no one was home. Not even his brother and sister who would usually be coming home by that time. Not having a key, he could not get into the apartment so he had to wait. By five o'clock, the neighbors living in the first floor rear apartment behind the delicatessen saw that he was still outside and took him in. They[3] gave him supper for which he was very grateful. His parents showed up a couple of hours later but offered no explanation.

Inside the house was a payphone the so-called "nickel telephone." Once a month a telephone man would come around, open up the box, and collect the nickels. All calls were a nickel in those days; this would translate to perhaps fifty cents in today's more inflated currency. A common refrain of the time was:

I never call my Sadie Cohn upon the nickel telephone; I leave expensive things alone.

At about this time Bernie's father brought home the new technology of the time. This was a wind-up standing RCA Victrola which played records. Thus, the sound of Caruso, Galli-Curci and others would then be heard through the apartment.

In addition, at that time, owning an "icebox" required the horse and wagon delivery of a fifty-pound block of ice by the iceman who brought it in using a large set of tongs. While the iceman was inside making his delivery, kids, Bernie included, used to climb into the ice wagon, pick up and suck on the ice chips scattered about on an often-dirty floor. When Bernie was seven or eight, one of his household responsibilities was to empty the tray underneath the icebox on a daily basis, otherwise it could overflow.

During the summer, Bernie recalled that this home was close to the Italian section and often goats owned by the Italians would get loose and wander into the area. These goats would then have to be retrieved by Italian youths. On one occasion, Bernie remembered that he had his sun hat stolen by one of these older Italian boys.

One winter, Bernie's father bought him a beautiful new sled, one of the famous Flexible Fliers. Unfortunately, Bernie had left it on the second floor back porch and after only one week, it was gone, stolen. He was not only heartbroken by the loss but also felt guilty in that he had been careless and irresponsible. Needless to say, the sled was not replaced.

Milk was delivered in glass bottles to the back doorstep. In the winter the milk would freeze and expand pushing the paper stopper out of the bottle 2–3 inches. Milk was not homogenized at that time and the cream would rise to the top.

Bernie's brother, Jack, was given violin lessons and his sister, Tena, piano lessons. But for some reason Bernie was not taught to play a musical instrument.

Bernie recalled sitting on his father's lap as he was having his evening meal and "suddenly" a coin would appear as if from heaven, signifying that the good Lord had blessed the family. Bernie would get these coins as gifts. Since he had no bank to store them, he decided to hide them between the white piano keys. However, once placed in there he could not retrieve them. His older brother and sister sensing a goldmine decided to take the piano apart and "requisition" the coins. One time Bernie woke up and caught them in the act. He did not take kindly to their "acquisition" and bitterly complained to his father when he came home from work. This was one of the few times that Bernie saw his father scold his older siblings. Needless to say, all the coins were returned to Bernie.

Around 1920, aged eight, when in the fourth grade, Bernie's intellectual abilities began to be noted by teachers. He was singled out and considered the brightest student of the fourth grade class at Lowell Grammar School on the Northwest side of Chicago. Part of this may have resulted from the fact that Bernie had comprehended some mathematical problem particularly well, which led to his fourth grade teacher having him explain it to all the other fourth grade classes. Bernie was quite pleased with this recognition.

Bernie had a fairly normal upbringing, probably fairly typical for the times and looked forward to going to school. Education was to play a major role in Bernie's life from that moment on.

Chapter 14

GROWING UP IN CHICAGO

In the years from 1920 to 1925, Bernie grew from a child into an adolescent. The move from a largely Jewish neighborhood to a Protestant and Catholic Southside area also influenced Bernie's development.

In 1921, as did so many other kids over the years, Bernie, now nine, had a paper route. These had to be folded and thrown up onto 2nd and 3rd floor porches; this provided a few cents of spending money.

At another time, Bernie and another boy happened to be playing baseball when Bernie threw an errant ball that broke a small windowpane. Although it seemed that no one saw the incident, Bernie was fearful of the consequences and told his mother. Not too long after that a neighbor came over and indicated that Bernie was indeed the culprit who had broken the window. It cost 25 cents to fix it. Nevertheless, his mother sensing that he felt remorse and had learned a lesson, decided not to scold him, a point that Bernie never forgot. In addition, being the third and youngest child and very well behaved most of the time, he tended to be the favored one.

Nearby was Tuley High School, which Bernie's sister, Tena, attended. Bernie's older brother Jack, being more technically inclined, went to Lane Technical High School.

Next door to Evergreen Avenue apartment where they were now living was another apartment building in which lived friends, a family by the name of Reif,[1] who also came from Skidel, Belarus. Mr. Reif was an ingenious carpenter. To save the nickel it cost to use the telephone, he hooked up a line with a bell at both ends between the third floor of his apartment and the second floor of the Sarnat apartment, which was directly opposite. A ring got an instant response if someone was home, which encouraged conversation that might not otherwise have taken place.

The Reifs had an only son, Louis, who was near Bernie's older brother Jack in age. They told Jack that Louis was going to study dentistry. In 1921 only one year of college was needed to enter the Chicago College of Dental Surgery. Since Jack had already one year of college at Crane Tech, they both decided to enroll together in the Chicago College of Dental Surgery.

Bernie also recalled that Jack played the violin at this time and organized a quintet under the auspices of the Peerless Athletic Club. They would practice in the living room. The quintet included Jack on violin, Fink on drums, Lavick on piano and two others on coronet and trombone. This group of five musicians would play for weddings and bar mitzvahs and earn a bit of money. Bernie was quite impressed with their performance.

One Sunday, sometime late in 1921, Bernie, now nine, woke up to find that his brother had brought home a little puppy which he placed on Bernie's bed to his delight. In the beginning, Bernie's mother was opposed to bringing any animal into the house but later she became attached to the mixed breed, now named Topsy.

On another afternoon, the whole family had been out; on their return, they found that the inside of the apartment had been turned "white." The dog had found a sack of flour and got his teeth into it and spread flour all over the six-room apartment. Bernie's mother, needless to say, "saw red." However, she loved the dog dearly so it was not banished. One of the saddest days was when the family moved again, this time to the Southside of Chicago (see below), and as animals were not allowed in the new apartment, Bernie had to give up the dog. However, Bernie's mother saw to it that the pet was well cared for by giving Topsy to some close friends of theirs. After the new move, Bernie's mother would make weekly trips back to manage the building on Evergreen Avenue and this allowed her to visit the dog.

During this period, a cousin of Bernie's mother, Lottie Silverman from Syracuse, New York came to live with them. She was no youngster and what led to that arrangement was never clear to Bernie. After several months, his mother introduced her to Max Rooth, the elder son of some family friends. Soon after, a joyous wedding was held in their apartment. It proved to be an excellent marriage with a lovely daughter born several months later.

While still living on the Northwest side of Chicago, a distant cousin who was an Orthodox Jew influenced the family to join his Synagogue. Bernie did not believe that his parents were that Orthodox, rather it was just the closest Synagogue to where they lived. In contrast, the move to the Southside ended their affiliations with formal Jewish organizations.

Moving to the Southside

In the summer of 1923, after about two years at the Evergreen Avenue location, the family moved again. This was a consequence of Bernie's father buying the drugstore at 6529 Blackstone Avenue (65th and Blackstone) and that resulted in a radical change in their living. His father and brother were commuting between the Southside and where they were living on the Northwest side. The store was open from eight in the morning until midnight, 16 hours a day seven days a week. With travel of 45 minutes to an hour one-way, it became imperative to move to the Southside of Chicago so as to be closer to the drugstore. The new six-flat apartment building was on East 66th Place, located about two and one half blocks from the drugstore. When they lived on the Northwest side they were in a largely Jewish community; Bernie went to Lowell grammar school where the students were all Jewish. Now they jumped across the tracks, so to speak, from the Northwest side Jewish community to a predominately Irish Catholic/Protestant neighborhood. Bernie's family was the only Jewish tenant in the apartment building.

Bernie recalled that almost all their friends on the Northwest side were from the old country; that is, either from Volkovysk or Skidel in Belarus, presumably mostly from the Skidel side. Among some names were the Lomes. He remembered them because of the puppy that he could not bring to the Southside. His mother had farmed it out to the Lomes. Once in a while when he would come back to the Northwest side he would visit the dog but the dog no longer remembered Bernie, which broke his heart.

Other family friends that Bernie recalled were the Goodmans who introduced Bernie to a death in a family, actually for the second time. The first time was around 1919 when his father's brother died in New York. His name was Israel Sarnat and all that Bernie recalled was that a group of men came over and prayed (see chapter 11) which meant little to Bernie since he had never met his uncle Israel. The second occasion was with the Goodmans who had become close friends of Bernie's family. Mrs. Goodman, who must have been in her mid-thirties, died quite suddenly in 1921. The mourning of the family made quite an impression on Bernie. The third death that Bernie was to face occurred in 1921 when an eight-month old cousin died. The fourth one was in 1938 when one of his father's sisters died.

The Goodmans son Sidney became a dentist, a year behind Jack in dental school. When Jack got married, Sidney Goodman was the best man at his wedding. So contacts were maintained.

Among other family friends were the Barths. Rifka Barth was a friend of Bernie's mother's from Volkovysk. She was a lovely, well-educated woman, Bernie recalled from visits to their home. Her husband was a bookbinder who apparently did some of his work at home. He also had a carpentry shop. While Bernie never quite understood what that meant, he would get little blocks of wood to play with and take home.

The Barths had three children and Bernie remembered when he would come over for a visit at the age of four that one of their daughters, Sara, who seemed rather "old," was always weaving wigs from human hair at home. She had dummy heads and would fit the wigs to them. Bernie, of course, had no clue what they were for. She was making those wigs for Orthodox women who shaved their heads and then wore a *Scheipel* or head covering. Apparently this was her introduction to the beauty business. Another brother, Hec, sold beauty equipment and other supplies. Eventually, together they patented mascara known as "dark eyes." This became a small item in the Sears Roebuck catalog but it paid off handsomely for them. The third Barth child, Sam, became a teacher at Crane Technical High School in Chicago. Bernie and Rhoda kept in touch with the Barths throughout the years. In fact, when they lived in California after 1955, the Barth brothers would come to visit them. They were a wonderful family.

Another family friend went by the name of Koppel; Bernie's family knew several members of the family. Bernie remembered that on a visit there, Mr. Koppel would be working in his shop at home making cigars. He would roll them and put them into a mold and then place 50 of them into a box. In the early 1920's they were popular items according to Bernie.

These were the family friends that Bernie knew as a child. But when his parents moved to the Southside these relationships were no longer sustained and they were eventually dropped.

Within the Sarnat family, however, a cousin's club was formed in the early 1930's and was called the B'nai Mayers Cousins Club. These developed into social gatherings during the winter dinner meetings followed by a summer picnic. It grew to some 60 or 70, including first cousins, their spouses and their children. A newsletter was also published quarterly by the Cousin's Club. In 1946 Bernie became president of the Club for a year.

Bernie also recalled that as a youngster his parents went to the Yiddish theater on some Friday nights. Rather than hiring a babysitter, they would take him along. He remembered the curtain being on a roll and coming down from the top and making a bang when it hit the stage. While he did not really understand anything of what was going on, he could gather that the essence of the play was usually something about domestic difficulties, the husband-and-wife having trouble. As a kid he would get a little upset as these were not happy relationships. But this was Yiddish drama and his parents seemed to enjoy it.

His mother would try to keep a semblance of a kosher home. So once a week she would travel to the Northwest side because they still owned the three-story building there; and she would check to see if everything was all right as well as collect the rents. In addition she would get some kosher meats and bring back a week's supply. This went on for several years until it became a burden to her. As the youngest, Bernie had a good relationship with his mother. He would point out the inconsistencies in her efforts to maintain a kosher home but she would just smile and let it go. Several years later his parents finally sold the three-story building. She took care of the financial aspects of the sale since Bernie's father was busy with the drugstore.

This move entailed another change of grammar schools. Bernie left Lowell in the fifth grade and continued in the fifth grade at Walter Scott Elementary School at 64th and Blackstone Avenue. The class that Bernie now attended had some thirty-five students, in which there was only one other Jew.

The locations were such that Bernie's home, his father's drugstore and his school, were within a three to four-block walk. Bernie evidently showed some maturity, as he was chosen as one of two boys of the 6th, 7th and 8th grades to be a senior safety patrol leader, responsible for the crossing of students at the intersections near the school. He continued to be a very good student and was always at the top of the class. With each grade promotion he was given due recognition.

Bernie's eighth grade teacher, Miss Dover, a strict disciplinarian, once compared Bernie with Calvin Coolidge, then President of the United States and told the class that she expected a great future for him. Although Bernie was pleased, he did not try to imitate Coolidge's famous aversion to speaking.[2] He delivered the class address at graduation (Fig. 11).

Bernie was acutely conscious that he was short in stature. At the beginning of the school year in September, everyone, boys and girls, had to line up, according to height for physical education.

Invariably, Bernie found himself at the tail end of the group. Only later in high school, he finally found that there were students shorter than he was.

Bernie, like countless others, also joined the YMCA from 1925 to 1926. He engaged in sports all year around and, in spite of being short, he was selected as leader of one of the four teams consisting of eight to ten boys. His team also managed to come out first in the intramural sports competitions for the year.

Bernie was a very conscientious, serious and excellent student, if somewhat naïve. For example, he noticed that other students were being "skipped" or double promoted and he was not. Only much later did he realize that they were already too old to be in the grade in which they had been initially placed. Some of the students pointedly reminded him that he was Jewish, and one or two were openly anti-Jewish and refused to have anything to do with him, leaving him quite hurt.

Some Saturday mornings, Bernie and one or two of his gentile friends would gather wooden and cardboard boxes and make a fire in an empty lot at Marquette Road and Stony Island Avenue, and there they would roast potatoes. They could hardly wait the 45 or 60 minutes until they were adequately cooked. Although charred, they were delicious.

After the move to the Southside, Bernie devoted no time to being an observant Jew — quite the contrary. After moving to the Southside his family no longer belonged to a Temple. Nevertheless, they thought that when Bernie became twelve that he should go to Hebrew School and prepare for his Bar Mitzvah.

Therefore, after school, Bernie took the El (elevated train) from 66th and Blackstone to the 58th and Prairie neighborhood, about a 30-minute ride. This was a heavily Jewish area. So every weekday right after grammar school, he would arrive at the Hebrew School at about 4:00pm for an hour of instruction. The teacher, known as a melamed, was wearing a dirty black kaftan (cloak), a long beard, with mucous draining from his nose, a ruler in his hand, and his lecturing occasionally interrupted with an inhalation of snuff.

This was all strange and foreign to Bernie and he instantly disliked it. To make matters worse, Bernie was not able to perform to the teacher's satisfaction; he was repeatedly rapped on his knuckles with the ruler. When he asked about what he was learning by rote, he was told: don't ask. This further turned him against this so-called learning experience. When he complained to his parents, they said to be patient and that he would get a better teacher later. After continued complaints over several weeks, knowing that Bernie was an excellent student in grammar school, his parents indicated that he would not have to return. So he would not have a Bar Mitzvah and would be able to return to the earlier routine of playing with his friends Walter Clark and George Brooks, after school.

Among some of his other activities was selling sachet, gum and other low-price articles door to door. These products would be advertised in children's magazines, and then shipped to children who would receive "points" for the items sold and the cash sent in. These points could be redeemed for various items one of which was a "hand run" primitive motion picture projector with a strip of film. Bernie would set up a white sheet to project the film and would also turn on music so he had sound with the visual experience. This gave him much amusement, but did not propel him to Hollywood.

Often when there was a wedding in the neighborhood the wedding party would throw pennies from a second or third floor porch, and watch the children below scramble for the "hot" coins. Also in the neighborhood there was the "Penny Store" which catered to children who would buy candies, small wax bottles with some ill-looking liquid to drink, and "sun slides," which with the use of proper developing paper when exposed to the sun would create a picture of a favorite movie star.

He and three or four other boys also formed the Red Dagger Club, which involved reading and trying to behave like Robin Hood. At the rear of one of the member's homes, they dug a "cave" and held meetings of a sort during the fall and winter. Roasting marshmallows was a major activity.

By this time (mid 1920's) this neighborhood was already somewhat in decline. While generally middle class, those more affluent were moving in a southeasterly direction toward the Southshore of Chicago; that is, south of Jackson Park (Fig. 6). The neighborhood, south of the University of Chicago, part of an area called Woodlawn where the drugstore was located, would decline further in the next fifteen or so years becoming an economically depressed area as poorer black people moved in and whites moved elsewhere.

Irish Catholics

Blackstone Avenue marked the dividing line between the middle class Irish Catholics on the east side and the lower class Irish Catholics on the west side. These two groups would play a role in Bernie's life as he was growing up. It was also some time afterwards that the infamous Blackstone Rangers[3] held forth in an old building dating from the Chicago World's Fair of 1893, which was located across the street from his father's first drugstore.

Bernie's family had now settled down in a predominantly Irish Catholic/Protestant neighborhood, with the drugstore at 6529 Blackstone Avenue. These lower class Irish Catholics could be distinguished from their better-off middle class cousins. Bernie maintained good relationships with members of both groups. The poorer Irish did not have lace curtains on the windows and reflected lower class standards. Bernie recalled, around 1923 or 1924, that instead of butter these Irish used Oleomargarine. At that time, it was against the law for the manufacturer to add yellow to the margarine to make it look more like butter.

The poorer Irish were engaged in a number of activities, some legal and many not so legal. Bernie became involved with a few of them. For example, they would help themselves to a case of strawberries that were displayed outside of a local market, and make off with them. The owner was never able to catch them red-handed. On another occasion, they would sneak into the back of the horse-drawn Ward's bakery wagon that would pull up to make deliveries. They would then swipe donuts or other pastry goods while the driver was making a delivery. They were also engaged in other "activities." One of these involved golf.

Located a few blocks away, Jackson Park contained both a nine and an eighteen-hole golf course. The fourth hole on the eighteen-hole course was a water hole. Naturally, many of the golf balls would routinely end up in the water. Around nine or ten at night, a group of three or four of the Irish boys, plus Bernie, would head for the water hole, strip, dive in and search for balls in the water. Being aware of which side of the golf course water hole the police might show up, they hung their clothes on the opposite side and thereby managed their escape. The balls would then be cleaned and sold. It was also at this time that Bernie learned to play golf as a left-hander with right-handed clubs — a driver, a brassy, a midiron and a putter. He played the nine-hole courses and once in a while the 18-hole courses. One can safely say that he was no Tiger Woods.

Another activity involved the Oakwood cemetery adjacent to the Illinois Central railroad located south and west at 67th and Kenwood Avenue. Again, at night, they would jump over the wall and go fishing in a beautiful pond, which contained large Japanese Koi. Any fish they caught were taken home to eat. They were clever and knew how to avoid the night watchman.

In another endeavor, they would use bee-bee guns to shoot pigeons. They would then head for an empty lot and the pigeons would then be prepared and roasted over an open fire. Bernie, who ran around with them, however, did not either own a bee-bee gun or partake in the pigeon meals.

Clearly, their anti-social behavior, branded as juvenile delinquency, could have led to a life in crime. They were driven to this behavior largely because of hunger. However, in this case the opposite occurred. One of the Irish boys, Eddie Stafford, turned out to be an outstanding high school football quarterback who went on to win all-state honors. He was also an excellent golfer. Another two, Frank Signor and Al Anderaggen were also outstanding golfers.

Once, while the Irish boys were in church on Good Friday, Bernie was waiting for them outside. When they appeared they promptly beat him up. The reason was that they had been told that Jews were Christ-killers. Although small, he could physically handle two, but not four of them. Subsequently, they once again became good friends.

Bernie also associated with another group of Irish Catholics who lived East of Blackstone Avenue near Jackson Park. These were the middle class Irish and they did not exhibit the anti-social behavior of the previous group.

Bernie made two close friends while in grammar school.[4] One was an Irish Catholic named George Brooks who lived next door and the other was a Protestant boy by the name of Walter Clark who lived across 66th Place. After school, the three of them would play touch football in an empty lot nearby. As George Brooks was much bigger than the other two, he would play on one side against the other two. All three were Boy Scouts and belonged to the Eagle patrol of troop #528 (see Chapter 15). Eventually all three graduated from grammar school and entered Hyde Park High School in February of 1926. Walter Clark joined a fraternity[5] open only to gentiles and that relationship began to cool to Bernie's dismay. On the other hand, the relationship with George Brooks continued and Bernie was sort of a mentor to George in that he helped him academically through high school. Later, Bernie, who had been working in a drugstore owned by one of his cousins,[6] gave up the job and recommended George for the position, for which he was quite grateful. George Brooks never went on to college. In 1933, with the repeal of Prohibition, George and Bernie celebrated by drinking alcoholic beer in what was now no longer a speakeasy at 53rd and Harper Avenue.

Jackson Park

Jackson Park played an important part in the social life of the community. After the move to the Southside of Chicago, Jackson Park also played a role in Bernie's life from the time he moved there in the early 1920's until the move from Chicago to California in late

1955. Jackson Park proved to be not only a wonderful recreational area but also was a source of knowledge to be explained later.

In the summertime of the years 1923–1925 Bernie used to go to the beach and walk across from Stony Island Avenue all the way to the lakefront, a fairly long distance. He could also take a special bus for a nickel, but rather than do that he saved the ten cent round-trip fare so that he could get a hot dog and spend a good part of the day at the beach.

Another aspect of Jackson Park besides swimming in the summertime was that one of the Boy Scout tests he had to pass was an examination on geography and he drew a map of Wooded Island. The north and south ends of the Island were connected to the main portion of Jackson Park by curved Japanese bridges and he remembered how intrigued he was by these bridges as a youngster. These bridges were the remains of the 1893 World's Fair when Jackson Park was developed. On Wooded Island there were Japanese teahouses; although they were closed but the outside exteriors were quite pretty.

Another aspect of Jackson Park was that at the north end, at the 56th Street border, there was a large deserted museum also from the 1893 World's Fair. Sometime in the 1930's, Julius Rosenwald had it renovated, a tremendous project. It subsequently became the Museum of Science and Industry, which still provides a wonderful educational experience.

Bernie remembers his time in Jackson Park well. While in high school he would walk from the high school across the Park to where he then lived on Yates. The path would take him past the yacht harbor and in the summer various people with their boats would moor them there. At that time, there were replicas of the three ships, the Santa Maria, Niña and Pinta that Columbus used when he first made landfall in the Americas in 1492. These were also remains of the 1893 World's Fair.

When Bernie was living on East 56th Street and attending medical school, after studying intensively for many hours he would need a break. He would walk over to Jackson Park and the Wooded Island, taking a bag of peanuts with him to feed the squirrels.

This would be some recreation for a half-hour to 45 minutes, and then Bernie would return to his books.

Also near the south end of Jackson Park, near the yacht harbor, there was La Rabida Hospital for sick children. This was staffed by University of Chicago physicians. Just north of 56th Street, adjacent to Jackson Park, was an area where Bernie would go swimming on hot summer nights in the 1930's after he would close the drugstore at midnight. A couple of the fellows and Bernie would go over to what was then known as the Point, a bunch of tremendous rocks irregularly placed as a break water, and it was rat infested. Bernie guessed that the rats scampered away when they arrived near midnight to go swimming off the rocks. It was somewhat treacherous but a great cooling-off place and everyone enjoyed it very much.

The region around the Point was redone in the late 1940's and carefully manicured and landscaped. Today the area is known as the Promontory, which has become a very popular place for people to watch the lake activities.

Jackson Park would again play a role in 1947 to 1955. At that time Bernie lived on Chappel Avenue which was a couple of blocks south of Jackson Park. On Sundays he would take his two children for walks and meet Rhoda's Uncle Julius and talk while the children would play along the way.

The Illinois Central

The Illinois Central suburban railroad was the transportation nerve center from Hyde Park, Woodlawn and the South Shore areas to downtown Chicago. In addition, it also served other southern suburbs of Chicago. In the 1920's, when Bernie lived at the 66th Place, the house was located about a block away from the railroad station. At that time steam locomotives were used to pull the trains. They would come by on a regular schedule; the train was efficient and reliable. In the 1920's it would emit smoke, cinders and a smell, which Bernie was well acquainted with. In the 1930's, the Illinois Central was electrified. The reliability of the railroad was a great strength for the whole community.

Rise and Demise of the Movie Palace

A separate aspect of Bernie's growing up years, like that of millions of his generation, involved going to movies. Bernie lived through almost all of the history of the movie industry. When Bernie lived at 2558 Iowa Street, at the time he was in the early grades of school, his mother would sometimes take him with her while going marketing on Saturday evening. One of the places they went to was the Banowitz Bakery, where in exchange for purchases, she would receive tickets to the Harmony Theater next door. This was a rather primitive, barren room, the seats were wooden and hard and as they would come into the room, the screen was empty without a curtain. Nevertheless, they would show silent movies. Up front would be an upright piano and a person would play the appropriate music for the movie on the screen. This movie house was on Division Street near Humboldt Park.

The next phase in motion picture theater development as seen through Bernie's eyes occurred when Bernie lived on Evergreen Avenue. This theater was on the other side of Humboldt Park. Bernie would walk along Kedzie Boulevard to North Avenue where the Biltmore Theater was located. This was a somewhat less primitive theater in that the seats were now semi-upholstered and there was a curtain covering the screen. When the movie began the curtain would open. On the program would be cowboy-and-Indian pictures as well as Buster Keaton and Charlie Chaplin comedies. One or two reel movies would be shown. Bernie preferred the latter. Also available, of course, were popcorn and candy bars. This was a nice way to spend a Saturday afternoon.

At about this time, Balaban and Katz had opened up the Central Park Theater on the west side of Chicago. This represented another major advancement in the development of movie theaters. One day Bernie's father took him all the way to the Southside of Chicago, to 63rd and Cottage Grove Avenue, to the newly opened Balaban and Katz's Tivoli Theater. This theater was quite grandiose; it seated about 1500 people, there were two or three balconies, the seats were upholstered and the aisles had rich carpeting. There was an open foyer several stories high with artwork, tapestries, etc., a bit of "culture," if rather ornate. The program was much more extensive and what was really novel was that it would usually change each week. In addition, it would begin with a current news reel — Pathé News. This was followed by a 10 to 15 minute program by the symphony orchestra, located in the orchestra pit, which would also play later during the motion picture presentation. Then came the stage production, the elegant curtain would open and there would be a popular band on stage. One of these was the Benny Krueger band with Frankie Masters, a popular singer at the time. After about 15 to 20 minutes of popular music and songs, this part of the program would end. Next, would come the principal part of the program, the silent movie with accompanying music. This total program, about three hours in length in the afternoon would cost about 25 cents. Additionally, there were formally dressed ushers to direct you to your seats in what was a large theater for the times. The upper balconies were less expensive.

In addition to the Tivoli Theater, on the Southside, Balaban and Katz also opened theaters on the Northside and the Westside of Chicago. They also opened several theaters in downtown Chicago. On State Street was the large Chicago Theater, on Randolph Street was the Oriental Theater, and subsequently across from the Chicago Theater they opened the State — Lake Theater. So Balaban and Katz had become a colossus in the movie theater industry of Chicago. They gained national importance and eventually developed a relationship with Paramount Studios in Hollywood, California. During this period the Marx Brothers (not related to the comedians) also developed several similar theaters in Chicago.

Then in the 1930's a revolution in the motion picture industry occurred — the introduction of sound. Eventually, the orchestras and the stage shows disappeared. After World War II when the Sarnats lived in South Shore in the late 1940's and 1950's, two theaters comparable to the Balaban and Katz theaters, the Avalon and the Capitol Theaters added gimmicks like clouds and skies with stars to their ceilings.

The final major change occurred toward the end of the 20th century when these large grandiose theaters were no longer in vogue and were replaced by multi-theater complexes consisting of a number of smaller theaters each with 100 or so seats. The next chapter picks up on Bernie's membership in the Boy Scouts and his ongoing education.

Chapter 15

BOY SCOUTS AND ON TO HIGH SCHOOL

While living at 1449 East 66th Place for the next four years, a number of events took place. One of which was that in 1924, at the age of twelve, Bernie was eligible to join the Boy Scouts. The troop was comprised of Catholics and Protestants with Bernie being the sole Jew. Here, he was welcomed into the group and rapidly progressed up the Scout ladder becoming a First Class Scout on April 24, 1925 and subsequently winning numerous merit badges.

The troop 528 was conveniently located about one block from where he lived. They met for weekly meetings at All Souls Church on Friday evenings from about 7:00 to 10:00 pm, in uniform. The group was divided into four patrols of about eight boys each. Bernie belonged to the Eagle Patrol and was made assistant patrol leader. The scout leader Edward Lalor, then about nineteen, was a student at the University of Chicago, and was considered to be a fine leader by Bernie (Fig. 9).

Once or twice a year, they would attend Scout rallies where they would compete against other troops such as Scout troop 519 of Scott School and troop 505, which had so many members that it was composed of four separate units. Temple Isaiah sponsored this group.

Boy Scout Summer Camp

In 1926, at age of 14, Bernie went to his first Boy Scout summer camp (Fig. 10). His sister Tena always felt that he was socially shy, too much of a "momma's boy" and suggested that he should become more acquainted with the "outside" world. At that time, she had finished high school and was working as a legal secretary. As she was now earning a rather good salary as well as contributing some of it to the family support, she was able to pay for Bernie's two-week Scout camp. The total costs included transportation by ship, food, lodging and various activities came to twelve dollars.

Bernie had never been away from home alone for so long a period so Scout camp Owasippe became a defining experience. Bernie and a few other Scouts from his troop 528 as well as a few hundred other Scouts took a steamer from Navy Pier in downtown Chicago traveling for eight hours (during which time Bernie got seasick) in a northeastern direction and finally docking at Muskegon, Michigan.

Bernie had to get used to new surroundings, to the several hundred new boys that were strangers as well as the strange food as his mother tried to keep kosher at home. He recalled that a cannon was fired at six in the morning as a wake-up call after which they headed toward the adjacent inland lake about 100 yards away, stripped to shorts to exercise and then took a nude dip in the lake. The water was not only cold but also the bottom was so muddy that once out of the lake the legs would be not only covered with mud but also contained blood-sucking leeches. Then off to breakfast where Bernie learned to eat and enjoy bacon and eggs.

Around this lake, there were three campsites with troops from other parts of Chicago, some from the Northside, some from the Westside and some from the Southside (which included members of Bernie's troop). These various campsites would engage in intramural competition.

Bernie lived in a tent with upper and lower bunks, with eleven other boys from different troops. They decided as part of their required camp competition project to cooperate and build a wooden bridge. After consulting in the library, they then dug a large hole and commenced to build the overlying bridge using logs. The group thought they had built a pretty good-looking bridge. Unfortunately, when the judges attempted to cross it, it sagged indicating that the engineering was more than a little suspect, which led to their disqualification.

At the end of the first week, they broke camp and for the next three days, groups of four would go out and forage on their own using knapsacks, blankets and a supply of food. They could go anywhere they wanted to using maps and compasses. They slept out in the open for two nights. They ended back in camp on Sunday afternoon and were glad to be able to sleep in their bunks again. It was a great exploring experience.

The Friday before the Scout camp broke up, they had awards night and to Bernie's surprise, he was given a leadership award. He was a second-class Scout at the time and evidently showed some leadership abilities. It was an extremely enjoyable experience for Bernie, one that stayed with him for the duration of his life.

Another feature of the Boy Scout experience that Bernie fondly remembers was the overnight weekend hikes away from home to nearby Palos Park in the forest preserves. This early Scouting aspect was wonderful. They packed knapsacks and took blankets, food and personal items. On Friday afternoon, leaving by streetcar and then following a three-mile hike, they arrived at camp Kiwanis. Although Bernie thought he was in excellent physical condition, about halfway through the hike he was perspiring and the load that he was carrying had become a bit too much. His good friend Wally Clark, who was no bigger although wiry, took Bernie's pack in addition to his own, the rest of the way. Bernie was much relieved and appreciative. Once in camp, they prepared the tents with their bunks for the night. The troop then gathered firewood and started the campfire (fire by friction). Dinner was prepared consisting of Hunter's stew, creamed rice, creamed onions, and rice pudding. Never did dinner taste so good! Bernie could still recall the details of the event some 78 years later. He learned various aspects of scouting in that two-day period, would return on Sunday afternoon comfortably tired and totally relaxed, having had a wonderful weekend learning about nature. Bernie participated in these weekend outings several times. However, with the start of high school and having moved away from the area as well as working in the drugstore left little spare time so Bernie had to regretfully drop out of the Scouts.

Hyde Park High School

Bernie attended Hyde Park High School at 62nd and Stony Island Avenues across from Jackson Park from February 1926 to June 1929. At this moment in time the school had a mixture of about 75% White and 25% Black, 65% Christian and 35% Jewish students. It was predominantly middle class.

By the time Bernie had started at Hyde Park High School, the family had been living at 66th and Blackstone. They moved again to an apartment at 7019 Michigan Avenue, which was close to the new drugstore at 69th and Indiana Ave (Fig. 6). During this time Bernie worked from 7 to 10pm, four evenings a week, at his father's and later at a relative's drugstores. While the family now lived closer to the drugstore, this now required a streetcar ride to Hyde Park High School.

A number of famous alumni from the school include Walter Eckersoll, an outstanding athlete and Amelia Earhart who came back to speak at one of the assemblies in the summer of 1928. The 1929 "Aitchpe" (standing for Hyde Park) yearbook was dedicated to her. Among other distinguished graduates from Hyde Park High School were Mel Torme, Steve Allen, Herb Alpert, as well as Paul Samuelson, a Nobel laureate who eventually ended up at MIT as Professor of Economics, after having been a student at the University of Chicago. Another famous alumnus was Martin Kamen, who went to the University of Chicago and then on to Berkeley. He was co-discoverer of radioactive isotope Carbon-14. However, it was Willard Libby who eventually received the Nobel Prize for the development of Carbon-14 as an archeological dating method.

So many alumni had left Chicago over the years that sometime before 1980 a West Coast alumni group was formed in Los Angeles.

There is a meeting every five years with an attendance frequently of over 700. As of 1990, 1277 people were listed as members. They have come from as many as 24 different States and some even from abroad. At the time of this writing California has 1048 members with 229 from out of the State.

A number of students from Hyde Park High School went on to the University of Chicago, which was nearby. For Bernie beginning high school entailed some major changes in his life. It was a time of transition. Whereas in grammar school he did very well in his studies with minimal effort, he now found the courses more demanding and required intensive study. With the help of his sister, Tena, during the first month of attendance, he made the necessary study adjustments. He did very well, graduating with honors and obtained not only early admission to the University of Chicago but also received advanced college credit for some of his high school courses.

The second major adjustment was social. He now found out in a different way that he was a Jew. As already mentioned in Chapter 14, his very good friend in grammar school and Scouting, Walter Clark, while in high school, had joined a Gentile fraternity, would no longer associate with Bernie. This was a devastating personal blow to Bernie. Nevertheless, during his freshman year in high school, he became acquainted with Philip Shaneding who later was also a pre-med and medical student at the University of Chicago with Bernie, as well as being best man at Bernie's marriage to Rhoda in 1941 (see Chapter 19).

Two others with whom Bernie became close friends with in high school were Herbert Kreisman and his friend Bernie Colby. Bernie met Herbert Kreisman in their first year algebra class and they competed for top honors in the class. They continued to take math classes including trigonometry where they also competed for top honors. Both joined the honors math club in which they were officers at that time. Herbert Kreisman became an engineer after attending the Illinois Institute of Technology. Bernie Colby, like Bernie, also eventually attended the University of Chicago and obtained a law degree there.

Rather than have lunch in the school cafeteria (only when it rained), Bernie and his friends would go across the street from the high school to Cook's Sandwich Shop located in the Tower Building. There they could get sandwiches for 5 cents and a drink for 5 cents. Alexander's restaurant on Stony Island Avenue just south of 63rd Street was too expensive. Lunch there was 35 cents! They were known as the 'hungry four'. After an evening of "carousing," usually at a private home "speakeasy," they would end up at the White Castle hamburger place (5 cents for one) and splurge by eating two or maybe three hamburgers, if they had the money.

So the four of them, Philip, Herbert and the two Bernies, became life-long close friends — all Jewish. They apparently shared much in common; their ethics, scholarship, and none of them dated girls in high school.

Thus, one of their bonds of friendship was their mutual agreement to have nothing — or at least as little as possible — to do with girls, misogynists at the mature ages of 14! To make it official they drew up a document on parchment vowing to never marry and signed it in "blood"! If one of them broke the vow, he would have to treat the others (with their dates) to a steak dinner with imported French champagne. They actually maintained the vows for more than a decade. As it would happen, Bernie Sarnat was the first to break that vow in 1941 at the age of 29 (see Chapter 19). With no money to speak of, he and Rhoda were able to treat the eight of them to steak dinners and champagne. Whether it was really French champagne, Bernie does not recall, but the total cost came to 24 dollars. Subsequently, all the others did get married. When the fourth one (Herb) finally got married, some ten years later (1951), the tab had risen to 250 dollars. Each had married a different type of woman. They were all wonderful and the four couples remained very compatible with each other.

Their friendship which began in 1926 lasted until very recently. Herbert Kreisman died in 1998, Philip Shaneding died in 2003, and Bernice Colby died in 2007, so only Bernie Sarnat remains alive. During these many years, the group of eight remained close and they would get together for one trip a year. They were fondly remembered by Bernie and included trips to the Canadian Rockies, Toronto, Montreal, and to New England for the changing of the leaves during autumn. They also included other scenic places as well, such as Aspen, Colorado, Santa Fe, New Mexico, and Brandeis University (Fig. 52) in Waltham, Massachusetts, Ashland, Oregon and La Jolla, California.

Chapter 16

UNIVERSITY UNDERGRADUATE YEARS (1929–1933)

When Bernie's father purchased the third drugstore at 57th and Blackstone in the May of 1929, the family was living in South Shore about four or five miles away. Most of the people in the area of the drugstore lived in lovely private homes, others in apartments. Many of these homes were beautifully described in a book by Jean Block.[1]

Across the street from the drugstore was the Harvard Hotel, a four-story building, a livable relic from the 1893 Worlds Fair, since demolished. On 59th St. between Blackstone and Dorchester Avenue was the three-story Del Prado Hotel, another distinguished building dating from the 1893 World's Fair. This building was replaced by the International House in the early 1930's, a residence for foreign scholars and students at the University of Chicago. A then relatively new multi-story exclusive apartment building, primarily for faculty members in the early 1930's, was the Cloisters at 58th and Dorchester Ave. Another building was the Blackstone Hall on the avenue by the same name, a six-story private dormitory for college and business women. Finally, at the east end of the Midway at 59th and Stony Island Avenue there was the Vista Homes Apartments, some 14 stories high. A number of faculty members also resided there. At the west end of the Midway was the famous Laredo Taft sculpture "The Fountain of Time."

In September 1929, the family moved to University Avenue (Fig. 6), which was just two blocks away from the University of Chicago campus, but seven blocks away from the drugstore. The family lived there from 1929 to 1931. In 1931 the family moved to Dorchester, which was only three blocks away from the drugstore so, this was much more convenient. Then in 1933 the family moved again, this time to East 56th street, which was now just around the corner from the drugstore. Bernie lived here[2] until he married Rhoda in 1941 (Chapter 19).

Bernie was always a curious youngster, although he never had any direct experience with research endeavors. His curiosity about scientific research was a major influence later when it became time to apply to a university. In a conversation with a good friend, Mortimer Wolf, Bernie mentioned that he wanted to go to the University of Chicago at which point his friend indicated that he was enrolling at Northwestern, why didn't Bernie want to go there? His friend also added that he wouldn't want to apply to the University of Chicago because they were basically interested in research. To which Bernie replied: "That's just why I want to go there!"

University of Chicago

Bernie was accepted at the University of Chicago with advanced standing and enrolled there as a freshman in 1929. It was the same year that Robert Maynard Hutchins became president of the University at the age of 29. Bernie's pre-med curriculum lasted the usual four years and he graduated in 1933 with a bachelor's degree and entered medical school (Fig. 12).

Bernie's intention was to first obtain a medical degree and then follow that with a dental degree. With this educational background, he planned to pursue a career in oral and plastic surgery. Already at the age of nine he had been greatly influenced by his brother Jack, who was enrolled as a dental student at that time and in some ways acted as a father figure to Bernie. His brother urged him to go into a dental specialty and Bernie, somewhat naively, followed the suggestions of his older brother.

Bernie's sister Tena wanted him to go to the University of Illinois, which was about 100 miles South in Urbana. She thought that it would be a good experience for him to be away from home, become more socially adjusted and join a fraternity. However, he chose to go to the University of Chicago, a scholastically more demanding university and continued to live at home.

Eventually, he did join a fraternity upon his sister's insistence, which was Kappa Nu. This fraternity eventually merged with Zeta Beta Tau, also a Jewish fraternity. At that time there were 30 fraternities on campus, of which seven were Jewish. Prior to this time, Bernie had never dated a girl, and as the fraternity had two social events a year, Bernie was forced to get a date. Since his dancing abilities were quite limited, he took some formal lessons at Teresa Dolan's Dance Academy at 63rd and Woodlawn Avenues. Bernie was a slow learner. It was while at this dance school that the book *Studs Lonigan* by Charles Farrel had come out. Bernie recalled that in the book the leading character met a young and pretty freshman girl from Hyde Park High and then developed gonorrhea! This made the opposite sex less attractive. Each June at commencement time there would be an inter-fraternity singing session in the evening. Each fraternity with its complete membership would march into Hutchinson Common and around the fountain singing one of their marching songs. It was a well-attended gala affair. He made a few very close friends in the fraternity, several casual friends and a few bitter enemies.

The fraternity tried to get Bernie to be more physically active so they urged him to try out for varsity wrestling. After class at about 3 pm, he would go to the gym and wrestle for an hour or two, get home by about 5:30 or 6 pm, have dinner and be so tired that he would fall asleep. He would wake then about midnight and try to study for a few hours before falling asleep again. This rigorous routine between working in the drugstore 30 hours a week, going to a university with high academic standards, wrestling, and other fraternity activities did not help Bernie's grades. Therefore, in his third year he dropped out of the fraternity and started to concentrate more on his studies. Although he did drop out of varsity wrestling, he continued with intramural wrestling, where he won the gold medal in his weight class two years in a row, making him all-intramural university champion. Regretfully however, Bernie did not have either the opportunity or the time to take advantage of the rich options that an educational institution like the University of Chicago and its student life had to offer.

In about 1932, during the depth of the Depression, Isadore and Fanny, Bernie's parents, had saved enough money to start building a summer home in Paw Paw Lake, Western Michigan. Until about 1955, the Bernie Sarnat family enjoyed vacations there during the summer. While in college and medical school, Bernie would stay there with some of his friends for several days between the school breaks. In 1958, with both of Isadore's sisters no longer living there and his family dispersed, the Paw Paw Lake cottage was finally sold.

Kindling of Research Interests

Since he had been working 30 hours a week in his father's drug-store, he was not able to partake very much in the activities on campus. However, in his third year (1931), his interest in research increased. During that year Bernie had decided to take an honors research course in physiology. Two Ph.D. graduate students were investigating the effects of secretin on pancreatic blood flow. Bernie became intrigued with this research area and became an integral part of that experimental group. Bernie spent several months with the group.

This research entailed the measurement of circulation in a dog, over a 10–12 hour span and required that the dog be "heparinized." One of Bernie's duties involved the measurement of 100 mg lots of heparin. This being 1931, heparin was not very well known and would not have been used medically. Today, heparin is widely used as an anticoagulant. A one-gram container of heparin cost about 12 dollars, which at that time was a lot of money. In the following quarter, he again spent time in the phys-iology department, where he learned a great deal about how to conduct research. As a result, Bernie became so engrossed in physiological research, that although his goal at the time was to study dentistry after medical school, he also seriously entertained the thought of pursuing a Ph.D. degree in physiology instead or possibly in addition.

While Bernie's laboratory courses (chemistry, physics, comparative anatomy, cytology, microbiology, etc.) as an undergraduate at the University of Chicago were demanding and necessary requirements for admission to the University of Chicago School of Medicine, he did manage to take other courses such as Philosophy, Cultural Anthropology, Astronomy, Economics, Psychology, German and Mathematics. Bernie remembered that in his physics class with about 30 students, one of them, Sidney Smith, would regularly fall asleep.[3] This student was bored because he was way ahead of the class. Nevertheless, he flunked and was not admitted to the University of Chicago School of Medicine. However, he was subsequently admitted to the University of Louisville School of Medicine.

Nevertheless, in spite of a leaning toward research, Bernie remained true to his initial set of goals, first medical school and then dental school. Bernie's choice of dentistry was influenced at an early age by his brother Jack. When Bernie was in the fourth and fifth grades of grammar school, his brother Jack, was going to dental school and he would tell Bernie about his famous professor who had an M.D., D.D.S., L.L.D. and other degrees. He was a world famous oral and plastic surgeon in his day, from the 1890's to the 1920's, by the name of Truman W. Brophy. Families from all over the world would bring their children to him in Chicago to operate for cleft lip and palate.

Chapter 17

ON TO MEDICAL SCHOOL AND BEYOND (1933–1937)

At the outset, it might be instructive to describe briefly how the School of Medicine at the University of Chicago developed. The University of Chicago was founded in 1892. The new University opened its doors on the Southside adjacent to the Midway where the 1893 World's Fair was held. The first president of the university was William Rainey Harper. He was a very dynamic individual who recruited an outstanding faculty, which became the basis for the new University of Chicago as a private university.

Interested in research, Harper did not want any proprietary schools at the University but he made exceptions for medicine, law and business. He also did not want either a school of engineering or a school of dentistry. In 1897, Harper expressed the opinion that he always wanted a medical school on the campus on the Southside. In 1898 Rush Medical College, which at that time was very well known throughout the United States and worldwide, agreed to affiliate with the University of Chicago. Rush Medical College was far better known than the University of Chicago. In 1901, the first two years of basic sciences were offered on the University's Southside campus and the last two years, the clinical years, were being offered by Rush Medical on the Westside of Chicago.

In 1923, the University decided to open its own medical school on the Southside as an integral part of the university and the Rush Medical-Presbyterian Hospital Group was offered the opportunity to join the university on the Southside. They declined this offer partly probably because an aspect of the new medical school was that it would be composed of full-time faculty. In other words, at Rush Medical there were physicians who were in private practice and only secondarily came to Rush Medical to teach. The University of Chicago philosophy was that they would be primarily teaching and carrying out research at the university on the Southside at their medical school there. The University School of Medicine on the Southside began its first full class in 1924. This was a rather new concept at that time and the Rush-Presbyterian group did not feel comfortable enough to accept this. As a result in 1939 the University of Chicago dis-affiliated from Rush Medical which was again left as an independent school. It subsequently affiliated with the University Of Illinois School Of Medicine as a Post-Graduate School.

When the new medical school was founded on the Southside, Dean Lewis was selected to be the first chairman of the Department of Surgery. However, he accepted an appointment at Johns Hopkins and, of course, went on to develop an illustrious surgical service there. Dallas B. Phemister was the next choice and he served as a distinguished Chair of the Department of Surgery at the University of Chicago for many years until his retirement. He was a very dedicated person. His life was really devoted to the medical school where he made major contributions. The third of the illustrious trio of surgeons from the Rush Medical School was Evarts Graham who established an outstanding Department of Surgery at Washington University in St. Louis.

Bernie started medical school at the University of Chicago in 1933 and did his first two pre-clinical years on the Southside as did the entire class of 100 students. Many students then left for Rush Medical. In 1934 Bernie was fortunate to be accepted in a class of about 35 students who stayed on the Southside. Here they had several hospitals locally, Albert Merrit Billings housed Medicine and

Surgery, Bob's Roberts housed Pediatrics, and Chicago Lying-in Hospital housed Obstetrics and Gynecology. Thus, they were able to do all of their training within the confines of the hospitals on the Southside and rotate through each of the services without having to go very far afield. In the latter part of the 20th century and into the 21st century the medical students tend to travel more around the city to different hospitals for their clinical training so that the old concept of having all the training under "one roof" apparently does not seem to be followed so much anymore.

Nevertheless, there were a few exceptions to the "one roof" rule even then. The Medical School had a service at the contagious disease hospital, which was on Western Avenue around 26th street as Bernie recalled. There they would go once a week for the various contagious disease studies. Archibald Hoyne was the director and a wonderful teacher and speaker. The only other time that they left the University for training was on the home obstetric delivery service.

Working While Attending Medical School

Bernie played a role in each of the three drugstores that his father had owned. In the first one, in the early 1920's, at 6529 Blackstone Avenue, he was in grammar school and became a delivery boy. He was charged to deliver the orders to the homes of different customers. In the second drugstore, at 69th and Indiana (1926–1928), he was in high school and he was assigned to sweep the floors and making gallons of chocolate syrup for the soda fountain for the sodas/sundaes. This required 3 or 4 gallons at a time and took a couple of hours. Bernie was fifteen at this time and also obtained an apprentice pharmacist license. By the third drugstore (1929), at 57th and Blackstone, he was a student at the University of Chicago. By his second year he had had general and organic chemistry as well as qualitative and quantitative chemical analysis and college algebra. So he was qualified enough to take the assistant pharmacist state board examination. He took the first part, the theoretical aspect and passed the first time. But he failed to pass the second part of the exam, the practical part taken some months later, which involved the making of emulsions, capsules, suppositories and powders, the first time. These procedures were already out of fashion at that time (1931) but were still required on the state board examination. He took the practical again and passed it making him now a full assistant pharmacist.

Among his other duties was washing the front large outdoor glass store windows with soap and hot water twice a week using a squeegee on a long pole. This was somewhat of an ordeal in the winter when alcohol and ammonia was added to the water to keep it from freezing. This also entailed mopping the tile floor inside the store after a snowfall, as customers would track in the snow and moisture dirtying the floor.

Therefore, in addition to going to the University of Chicago full-time, he also worked Friday from 6:00pm to midnight, closing the drugstore, and Saturday and Sunday from 12 noon to midnight. In addition, he had to cover for the temporary absence of the fully registered pharmacist. So at seventeen, working thirty hours a week, he received fifty cents an hour salary, which he used to pay his personal expenses and those at the University of Chicago. Because of limited funds he was not able to buy all of his textbooks and had to rely on the limited resources of the library.

By working all the time, Bernie supported himself through college and eventually medical school. Bernie's pre-clinical years of medical school were very demanding of his time. The question was always where to direct his limited energies for study while being sleep-deprived and physically and emotionally drained. The effects of this lack of sleep on students can be demonstrated with an example in one of the classes of 100 students. Projection of the slides in this particular class was carried out by a paid student who was clearly sleep-deprived. As the instructor asked for the next slide, nothing happened. "NEXT SLIDE PLEASE!" "Will someone please wake up the projectionist!"

In the summer of 1933, Bernie organized a party for his medical student friends with their dates (about 20 to 26 people) to spend a day on the Jack-Ellen, a two-masted yawl, about 40 feet in length. They would sail along the shore of Lake Michigan, go swimming, and observe the World's Fair while having lunch on-board. This proved to be a very pleasant and highly successful relaxing day. Consequently, Bernie repeated it again in 1934 as the World's Fair was continuing for another year. In addition, also in 1934, he organized a one-time "beer party" at his home for his fellow medical students.

Having to work at the drugstore Bernie, regretfully, was not able to take advantage of all the numerous activities available at the University of Chicago. However, during the last year at the medical school, which entailed the "grand finals" (oral, written and practical) he asked to stop working at the drugstore so that he could focus more on his studies. From then on, Bernie never worked in the drugstore again.

First Two Years of Medical School

As Bernie was finishing his second year of the basic sciences in the summer of 1934, the night before he was supposed to take some of his final examinations, he experienced difficulty and pain in swallowing. The right side of his face was tender and swollen. By the morning, he was supposed to go in for his final examinations. He had been up all night in extreme pain, could not swallow, so he went to student health. There they made the diagnosis of adult mumps. As a result, of course, he could not take his final examinations and was admitted to Billings Hospital. They had a two-bed contagious disease isolated center and Bernie occupied one of those beds. Not only did he develop parotitis (non-purulent) with acute severe pain, but he also developed adult unilateral orchitis as well, a swelling of the testicle, a relatively rare occurrence in adult mumps. So now he was in really acute pain and a very unhappy person. However, he did serve as a great teaching example for the students to see an adult patient with mumps and orchitis so that may have helped pay his hospital bill, although he was not sure. After several days in the hospital he was discharged but he was quite exhausted physically and weak. So he went up to his folks summer home in Paw Paw Lake to recover for another week or two.

With regard to the final examinations he had missed, he had already been excused from biochemistry because he had done so well. In physiology he was also excused but he had to take the pharmacology examination which of course he did pass and so in September of 1934 he was able to start his clinical work.

Last Two Years of Medical School

The first service Bernie had was obstetrics and gynecology and two experiences there in particular made quite an impression on him. He was on the service for delivering babies in the hospital and one of the patients that he was monitoring was a woman who already had two children and was in about her eighth month of pregnancy waiting to go into labor. This woman had a rheumatic heart which had decompensated. The doctors knew about this at the time she first came in for prenatal care and they advised that she should have the fetus aborted because not only would the process of going through pregnancy and labor be difficult, but also raising a third child would be just too exhausting for her. This patient was Catholic and the Church would not approve the aborting of the fetus. So the doctors did the best they could to carry her into labor.

At this critical juncture Bernie, as a student, was involved in the care of this patient and found that she was going into heart failure. The question then arose whether they should destroy the infant now and save the mother's life or allow the mother, at great risk, to go through labor to deliver the baby. They were not sure that they could bring either a live baby or a live mother through the delivery. The priest refused to permit the abortion of this infant and so she was carried on into labor. No sooner had she delivered the baby that she went into total heart failure and died. A dead baby was delivered! This experience had a tremendous impact on Bernie with respect to the socio-economic-religious effects of pregnancy, especially as a human being.

Another incident that remains sharply etched in Bernie's mind to this day some 70 years later was when he went on the home delivery service during Christmas vacation of 1934 for about 10 days. The students had a medical bag packed by the hospital with all the necessary equipment. This service was limited to women who already had one baby and this was at least their second pregnancy. As far as the prenatal care had determined, it should be a normal delivery. So on Christmas Day 1934, Bernie took a streetcar with his medical bag in hand and ended up on the Southside of Chicago in the largely black area. It had snowed that day and was moderately cold. When he arrived at the appropriate building and knocked on the door, a woman greeted him and he was taken aback because there was a rather tall, stately, and very attractive Caucasian woman who was obviously pregnant. She admitted him into her apartment and he obtained the information that was needed to set things up for the eventual delivery. Bernie examined her and had everything prepared. She did not appear to be in active labor so this delivery would probably take several hours. They were instructed to have a pot of water boiling and newspaper. It was found that old newspaper would be sterile and could be placed under the patient prior to delivery. Bernie glanced around the apartment and saw that there was a wonderful library of books including literature and he could not quite comprehend what this white woman was doing in the black neighborhood with a library that was so outstanding. During this time, a two-year-old black girl, her daughter, came in to say hello.

After an uneventful delivery the mother was given two aspirin tablets for pain and some ergot to help contract the uterus. Bernie also suggested drinking a quart of milk a day but the mother said she did not have enough money to buy milk, which was nine cents a quart. With Bernie's limited income, he gave the mother eighteen cents for two quarts of milk. After several similar incidents, he had to stop his philanthropy.

Bernie subsequently learned from the patient that she had met her husband at the University of Michigan where they both had been students. The reason her husband was not home was that he was the leader of the black communist movement in Chicago and he was out giving talks. It turned out that she was the daughter of the Chief Justice of the Supreme Court of Michigan, so all in all that day proved to be quite an experience.

One of the technical terms in obstetrics is a breech delivery, where the feet come out first rather than the head. This is known as a Frank breech. One of Bernie's fellow medical students who was feeling pretty good, decided one day to use the hospital calling system, a loudspeaker system throughout the hospitals. He called in to the operator and asked if she could page Dr. Frank Breech. So over the system one heard her paging Dr. Frank Breech. Of course the medical students thought this was a great prank. No one found out who actually did it.

While Bernie was doing his clerkship in medicine, the pharmacist clerk, Carl Maether, in his father's drugstore, had severe hemorrhaging from the stomach. When he was just out of Pharmacy School, he had worked for Bernie's father in the first and second drugstores. Bernie's father and Carl had a wonderful father-son relationship. Carl was very devoted to Isadore. When Carl suddenly developed this spontaneous gastric hemorrhage, he was rushed to Billings Hospital, given a series of transfusions and eventually the bleeding stopped. He was then placed on an ulcer regime and put on what was then known as the Sippy Diet, the name of a famous gastroenterologist of the day (This was of course years before the discovery of the cause — the bacterium *H. pylori*). This was a regimen of antacids used to neutralize the acids of the stomach. He recovered from that and came back to work but a few weeks later he hemorrhaged again. This happened several times. During this period when he was unable to work, Bernie's father paid his full salary. But after a few months, he had to hire another pharmacist in the place of the one who was now sick. After another few months his father had to, regrettably, cut the salary in half and eventually he no longer could take the financial burden. This was in 1934/1935 in the height of the Depression days and so Carl was transferred from the regular service to the ward service where there was no financial responsibility.

So while Bernie was on the medical service, he looked after his pharmacist friend and clerk, talked with him, helped him with his personal needs, and would shave him frequently too because he could not afford to pay for a barber. But, eventually, regrettably, he had another hemorrhage and died.

At that time the University gastroenterology service had brought over a Dr. Rudolph Schindler from Germany who had developed a rigid gastroscope, an instrument that could be passed down through the mouth into the stomach to study what was going on. The patient had to be anesthetized for this procedure. It was a really severe ordeal for the patient, let alone the doctor. Today, a flexible gastroscope is used, so it is a very simple procedure, and not only is the flexible gastroscope passed down but it includes a camera, which take pictures simultaneously.

Like many medical students, Bernie found that as one studies diseases, one begins to identify closely with the patient and at times thinks that one is experiencing them as well. In fact, when he was on the pediatric service and took care of children with diarrhea he also developed diarrhea. Consequently, Bernie felt that maybe he was getting an ulcer while on the medical service. When he was on the surgical service he thought he was getting a cancer of the bowel, which ironically he eventually did, in 1961 (see Chapter 27). No, he did not develop a pseudopsyesis when on the obstetric service.

In June 1936, having finished medical school and planning to go to Los Angeles for his internship, Bernie learned that transport companies in Chicago were interested in people who would drive new automobiles from Chicago to Los Angeles. The company would pay for oil changes but not for gasoline. They also included insurance. The car had to be delivered in Los Angeles within seven days. Bernie signed up for this and put a notice on the University of Chicago student bulletin board looking for students willing to share the trip expenses. Two students who were residents of Los Angeles immediately responded and agreed to share all driving expenses. One student was the son of the Dean of Pasadena City College. On the way they stopped off at Grand Canyon, Bryce and

Zion National Parks. As they approached Las Vegas, the other student who was Japanese, asked not to go into the motel when they registered for the night's lodgings. Little did Bernie realize that anti-Japanese sentiment was already strong in the mid-1930's. They reached Los Angeles uneventfully on the seventh day. Bernie delivered each of his two passengers, went on to the county hospital to discharge his belongings, and then delivered the automobile as promised. This turned out to be a wonderful trip on Route 66 in 1936.

Medical Internship

Having finished medical school at the University of Chicago, Bernie interned at the Los Angeles County General Hospital for a year (1936/1937). This was his first extended-time experience away from home (Fig. 13). He enjoyed the year, both medically and socially. Rhoda, Bernie's future wife was living in Beverly Hills at the time and attending UCLA. She, of course, did not exist as far as Bernie was concerned and it would have been extremely unlikely that they would have met in Los Angeles.

He started the internship in June 1936 at 24 years of age. Ten days before the formal internship was to start, they needed an intern to attend in the Infected Gynecology Ward. Bernie did not know what that particular Ward represented. But he soon found out. At that time LA County General Hospital had about 3000 beds with 2400 occupied with patients. One of the small wards was Infected Gynecology with about 30 patients. These women, some no doubt "ladies of the evening," had attempted abortion and in the process developed some sort of infection. So, when Bernie, the very young looking new intern walked into the Ward in his new white uniform, he was received with whistles from the patients who quickly realized that he was a novice doctor. Bernie was so embarrassed that he blushed, turned on his heel and ran out. Later, having overcome his embarrassment he began his prescribed duties.

The internship was unusually good according to Bernie, particularly because of the large patient population. This was quite a contrast from the small patient population in medical school. He had rotations (services) in medicine; dermatology; anesthesiology; general surgery; ear, nose and throat and oral surgery; cancer surgery; infectious diseases; and obstetrics and gynecology. When Bernie had a free evening, he would spend time in the admitting room to become acquainted with the wide variety of medical problems coming into the hospital.

To his surprise, he learned that there were two services: Doctors of Medicine (Unit I) and Doctors of Osteopathy (Unit II). They were separate and distinct. However, problem cases were sometimes sent from Unit II to Unit I.

Bernie also learned that the Seventh Day Adventists had a Medical School with a number of its graduates as interns. Consequently, the doctor's dining room served two diets — the regular one and a vegetarian one that was quite good and Bernie would eat it from time to time. The living quarters were like a hotel with the hospital just a few years old and not yet fully occupied.

During the year, he managed to see some of the sights of greater Los Angeles. He went to the Hollywood Bowl (Midsummer Nights Dream, premiere with Mickey Rooney), Lake Arrowhead, Palm Springs, Santa Anita racetrack, Catalina Island, the gambling ship, a movie premiere at the Cathay Circle (The Good Earth), swimming in the ocean, deep sea fishing, etc.

To relieve the monotony of hospital food Bernie, with some of his fellow interns, would occasionally eat out in a decent restaurant. Another highlight was visiting Aimee Semple McPherson at the Angelus Temple on Friday night which was "healing night." About 1500 were in the audience. Bernie wanted to see how she "healed" members. Being a skeptical and objective medical student, he was not impressed with the "revelations." He concluded that most of them were hysterics. He was impressed however, with the way Aimee McPherson, beautifully gowned with fancy jewelry, instructed the audience as the collection plates were passed with: "I don't want to hear the tinkle of the coins. I want to see the flutter of dollar bills." It is important to realize that this was in the depths of the Depression.

How did Bernie manage all of the above financially? He originally received $10 a month salary. His first paycheck was $9.10. He went to the front office and asked for his missing 90 cents and was told that it was going into his pension plan. But he said: "I'm only going to be for a year"; nevertheless, he never did see the "missing" 90 cents each month. In addition, his father would send him $10 a month. Lastly, every three months he was able to give a blood transfusion for which he received $25. So in one way or another Bernie managed to get along.

When he completed his internship in Los Angeles, it was time to start the second part of his program; namely, getting a dental degree.

Chapter 18

UNIVERSITY OF ILLINOIS
(1937–1940)

W hile in Los Angeles, Bernie decided to explore the possibilities available for the study of dentistry, not so much for the technical aspects, but more for the biological ones. This led to the University of Southern California (USC) Dental School. At this time, the University of California at Los Angeles (UCLA) had neither a dental nor a medical school. While being interviewed by the USC dental school dean (Bernie likes to think of it as the opposite — that is, he was interviewing the dean), he soon discovered that the dental school prided itself on producing technically proficient dentists who excelled in the manual arts of the craft but knew less of the underlying biology. Clearly, this was not Bernie's goal as he was primarily interested in the biological aspects of dentistry. Bernie then decided to leave Los Angeles and return to Chicago.

But before Bernie left to return to Chicago, he stayed for an extra six weeks, and took and passed the California Medical State Board examinations. He chose to be accredited in California because he thought he might want to return to California to practice in the future, especially considering that in Chicago, Bernie suffered from allergies and asthma from May to September, and had had no such problems during his one-year internship in Los Angeles.

Bernie's brother Jack proposed that he drive from Chicago to Los Angeles to pick him up. Jack, Bernie Colby and Sidney

Goodman arrived soon after Bernie had taken his Medical State Boards. After a week of pleasure and sightseeing in Los Angeles, the four drove up to San Francisco and traveled over the newly opened Golden Gate Bridge, on to Yosemite National Park and through the treacherous Tioga Pass and Yellowstone National Park on the way back to Chicago.

Applying to Dental School

Interestingly, when Bernie returned to Chicago in August 1937 from his internship in California, he indicated to his parents that he was enrolling in another course of study, this time leading to a dental degree. His mother was aghast and said: "But you are a doctor already!" Bernie suspects that his older brother Jack, now a practicing dentist for 12 years, had talked to their parents and prepared the way.

In August 1937, the same month in which he had returned to Chicago, he went over to see Dean Logan at the Chicago College of Dental Surgery,[1] later affiliated with Loyola University. This was the same school his brother, Jack, had earlier attended. He told the dean that he was not only interested in going to dental school but also wanted to do research and teaching. Dean Logan, a rather smooth and diplomatic person, patted him on the back and said: "Doctor Sarnat you are accepted to the dental school class starting next month and we will see about your teaching and research." However, this was just not a firm enough commitment for Bernie.

As planned, Bernie then went to Northwestern University School of Dentistry, where he was interviewed by Doctor Arthur Black[2] who also indicated that he could be admitted to the dental class the following month, but again did not receive any assurances that he would be allowed to do any teaching or research. So at this point, none of the dental schools at which Bernie had interviewed had satisfied his needs. Each had tentatively offered him something, but nothing, besides admission to the dental school, that was really substantial.

The fourth school that Bernie wanted to interview was the University of Illinois College of Dentistry, located on Harrison

Street on Chicago's Westside, because he knew of the reputation and the accomplishments of Dr. Schour who was there. Dr. Isaac Schour had obtained a bachelor's degree at the University of Chicago, a dental degree from the University of Illinois, and then went on to obtain a Ph.D. in anatomy from the University of Chicago. This was at a time (1937) when Schour was considered to be one of the foremost, if not *the foremost*, biological researcher in dentistry in the United States. A friend of Bernie's family, Dr. Louis Reif,[3] also knew Dr. Schour intimately and strongly urged Bernie to apply.

Bernie was first interviewed by Dr. Frederick B. Noyes, the Dean of the Dental School, a wonderful gentleman who put his arm around Bernie and said: "We want you very much at the University of Illinois and I want you to talk with Dr. Schour", which was exactly what Bernie wanted. In fact, Bernie had actually already set up an appointment to meet with him.

Bernie then went up to see Dr. Schour in the old dental building, at that time a decrepit wooden structure. He had a great interview. Dr. Schour was a wonderfully warm and understanding person. He had done basic research on teeth, the endocrine glands, as well as on vitamins. At 37, he already had an international reputation. Bernie walked into his lab and noticed the numerous lab benches and cages on the side with white rats. He also noticed that some of the resident gray rats were also on the outside of the cages. Once into his office, he noted the roll top desk heaped high with correspondence, scattered papers and books. One look at the rather busy (one might say messy) surroundings left Bernie in a doubtful state. But Schour gave him a cheery hello and sat him down for a chat, which quickly dispelled any doubts. As Bernie outlined his interests, Schour assured him that he was definitely wanted and that he would have a teaching position in histology (Fig. 27). Moreover, they would pay all the tuition and provide the dental instruments and material such as the gold for fillings. However, they could not pay a salary.

Therefore, the offer that Dean Noyes and Dr. Schour gave Bernie was that: (1) yes, they would give him a teaching position as an assistant in histology, and (2) yes, he could be registered as an advanced dental student, and (3) yes, he could register in the graduate school for a master's degree, allowing Bernie to pursue the research aspect. Now Bernie had the opportunity to really get involved in research in a way that he had not been able to do previously.

University of Illinois

While a student at the University of Chicago, Bernie had been working 30 hours a week at his father's drugstore to pay for tuition and other expenses. While he enjoyed the unusual group of customers and the University of Chicago faculty and others that frequented it, he realized that medical school was also a full-time endeavor. He then told his father that while he greatly appreciated the opportunity to work in the drugstore all these years, he wanted to be a 'free agent' so to speak. Therefore, in 1935, in his last year of medical school, Bernie permanently stopped working there. He was replaced with another clerk.

While in dental school at the University of Illinois, he lived at home with his parents on the Southside of Chicago, so room and board was free. To make his first class at 8:00 am, Bernie would have to get up at 6:30 am and take the elevated train to the Westside where the Dental School was located, a trip of 45 minutes or longer in winter.

Sometimes Lewis Robbins, whom Bernie knew from High School and the University of Chicago, would pick Bernie up in his big outdated "clunker" of an automobile at 7:30 am after his one hour psychiatric session with Roy Grinker M.D. and for 10 cents would drive Bernie to the Westside Medical Center where he attended Rush Medical College. Robbins subsequently held a top position for many years at the Menninger Psychiatric Clinic in Topeka, Kansas.

In 1938, Bernie's father and his brother Jack, realizing how hard Bernie was working, surprised him with a present. They had put $650 together and bought him a brand new Plymouth. It was just about the cheapest car available. It came with neither a radio nor a heater. While the former was not critical, the latter was, if you are going to spend winters in Chicago. Now Bernie could get to the University in about 30 minutes rather than close to an hour. That was a big help and Bernie was most appreciative.

Nevertheless, Bernie still needed money to make ends meet. Although he was able to practice medicine in California, he never intended to go into the general practice of medicine. His mind was instead focused on a career in surgical practice, teaching and research. Since he had passed the Illinois Medical State Board examinations, he could practice in Illinois as well. Thus, he was able to get a position with the Work Project Administration (WPA), allowing him to earn a bit of extra money to live on. The work entailed making house calls at the rate of $1.50 for each patient. He would go by streetcar with his medical bag making house calls. Later, when he drove the Plymouth, he had much more mobility and this allowed him to make his house calls with less difficulty, although having to pay for gasoline was sometimes a challenge at 0.11 cents a gallon.

Research Beginnings

Bernie began his dental school education at the University of Illinois in August of 1937 in the three-storey wooden, rat infested, firetrap of a building on Harrison Street. Just before Thanksgiving the dental school moved to the then ultra modern new 13-storey dental building at 808 South Wood Street. Initially when Bernie accepted the appointment, he was totally unaware of the contemplated move to the new building. The entire 10th floor was the teaching laboratory. On the 11th floor, Bernie had his histology office and research laboratory, which he shared with Fred Herzberg, a dentist interested in the biologic aspects of dentistry. They became very close friends. Although, their research interests were somewhat different, they shared much in common. Fred had a Carnegie fellowship of $1500 a year. Furthermore, he was of great help to Bernie in some of the technical aspects of the dental school training. This friendship was renewed in 1955 in California later with Fred's appointment at the UCLA Dental School.

In the laboratory there were five or six students working on their Masters and a few on Doctor of Philosophy degrees. Several of them were teaching assistants in the histology course for the first-year dental students. One had a number of diverse talents such as cutting hair for 25 cents. Bernie took advantage of the excellent service.

Collaborative work was done with the department of Pediatrics. Henry Poncher, M.D. was chief and Julius Richmond was in his department at that time. He is now Professor Emeritus of Social Psychiatry at Harvard Medical School.

On Monday at noon, Dr. Schour would invite prominent scientists to give what were outstanding weekly seminars. This was a brown bag lunch. Every Saturday afternoon Schour would supply the lunch for the various graduate students and teaching assistants for a general get-together in discussion and review of what was going on in the department.

William Winn was the photographer for the department and was kept very busy with their research efforts. Gertrude Everett was the departmental secretary. She was a very hard-working devoted Daughter of the American Revolution spinster. Apparently Bernie was one of her adopted boys because when he was nominated for full membership in Sigma Xi she was aware of this and proudly presented him with the key. This of course was a very pleasant surprise for Bernie. She did all of the typing of Bernie's manuscripts and in particular the one that was extremely difficult to type and was awarded the Joseph A. Capps award. Francis Schwab was the technician and did the histologic work for Bernie, particularly on yellow phosphorus and hibernation (discussed later). The final non-professional member in the department was Emil Matt who did general service and particularly saw to it that the luncheon was taken care of on Saturday afternoons as well as other "repair person" errands. Bernie became his family doctor and at one time took care of his young son who was quite ill. Bernie made the diagnosis of diphtheria and gave the needed anti-toxin and miraculously, the seriously ill child improved. Matt was indebted to Bernie and in return would service his 1938 Plymouth and also do other favors.

At the end of each academic year in June, the histology department would hold a picnic. Bernie's brother, Jack, had a modest one-room cottage at the Indiana sand dunes (Miller, Indiana, which was about 35 miles east of Chicago). The group would gather on a Sunday morning in June at the drugstore at 57th and Blackstone since this was on the way. In 1940, Esther Schour noticed that Bernie did not have a date for the picnic and asked if he would like to meet a very nice girl named Rhoda. He said yes and finally got around to calling her one year later, rationalizing that extenuating circumstances such as him being on call at the hospital, deeply involved in research and most importantly, not having any money to pay for a date, accounted for the time lapse (see Chapter 19).

There were several nationally and internationally known faculty members at the Dental School. Besides Isaac Schour and Dean Frederick B. Noyes, there were also Alan Brodie, head of graduate orthodontics, and Stanley Tylman, head of crown and bridge. Tylman was also the personal dentist of Juan Peron, dictator of Argentina at the time. Another member was J. Roy Blayney who had just left the University of Illinois to become the first head of the Zoller Clinic at the University Of Chicago School Of Medicine. He headed up an important project studying the use of fluorine for dental health. Another faculty member was Maynard Hine who left to become Dean at the Indiana University School of Dentistry. He eventually became President of Indiana University.

Dental school turned out to be an extremely busy time for Bernie. He not only had to keep up with his dental classes, but also with his responsibilities in graduate school and with being a faculty member. In the morning he would take courses with the first year students. In the afternoon he would assist and teach histology. As Bernie recalled the students were confused. Who was this fellow, Sarnat, a student with us in the morning and our teacher in the afternoon? The word soon got around that he was a bit unusual as an advanced student who had already obtained a medical degree. He was wearing two hats, so to speak. As a student, he was required to carve a set of teeth in wax at three times normal size. This would take four to six hours per tooth. Some of Bernie's medical colleagues would tell him that they had removed several gallbladders and appendices in that time. They questioned his goals.

Bernie was now engaged in a very intense research program over these three years (1937–1940). He was working seven days a week, sometimes 24 hours a day. Some of the experiments lasted over a 24-hour period requiring him to sleep in the laboratory. His interest was primarily in bones and teeth. This led to visits to the laboratory of Charles Huggins (Nobel Laureate) at the University of Chicago Medical School, who was also interested in bones and teeth at that time. Bernie initiated collaborative studies at Rush Medical College and the University Of Chicago School Of Medicine, dealing with the effects of yellow phosphorus on growing bones (tibia, base of the skull) and teeth. Another study was concerned with the decelerating effects of hibernation in growing teeth. In addition he began a long-term study of the teeth as recorders of systemic disease.

The study of teeth as recorders of systemic disease led to the first paper that Bernie published.[4] That long-term experiment initiated in early 1938 involved both clinical medicine and basic science. In 1939, this work won the Joseph A. Capps Prize offered by the Institute of Medicine of Chicago. The competition for the Capps award was open to any graduate from any one of the six medical schools in Chicago, for research conducted within a five-year period after graduation. This was the first time that a dental subject had won this medical prize. It was considered a highly coveted award, which led to instant recognition and represented the beginning of his well-known research career. In addition, based on this research, Bernie also received the Frederick B. Noyes Award given by the University of Illinois College of Dentistry.

Bernie was invited to present this work before the University of Chicago Medical Alumni Association in June of 1940 at the annual program for the Medical School reunion. In the audience was

Anton J. Carlson, Professor and Chairman of the Department of Physiology. He was a very clear thinker and questioner and raised some pertinent questions. This time Bernie was not the student but the expert and handled himself very well. At that time, he was elected vice-president of the Medical Alumni Association.

The projects on the effects of yellow phosphorus on bones and teeth and hibernation proved to be very productive studies and represented some of the earliest basic research for Bernie. Material for the hibernation project consisted of gophers captured on the University of Wisconsin-Madison campus. There was a state bounty of 25 cents each on these gophers because of their status as pests. The lab paid students 25 cents in addition to the 25-cent bounty for these specimens. There were several interesting experiences. The experiment was started in August and to place the gophers into hibernation there was a large walk-in refrigerator held at about 2 to 5°C. When one went in to check on the gophers during hibernation, it was found that the warmth of the hands would awaken them so they had to put on gloves. In addition, to keep warm, Bernie and colleagues had to wear coats, hats, and earmuffs.

Each gopher was placed in a separate cage. The gophers would wake up every two to three days. In one instance, the cages were too close to each other and one of them apparently had put its leg into the cage next to it and when it woke, all the flesh had been eaten off the extremity. This was an example of bloodless surgery; that is, anesthesia by refrigeration. The purpose of this experiment was to determine the effect of hibernation on dentin apposition. A calcium specific vital stain, alizarin red, was used. It was found that the rate of dentin apposition was decreased by as much as 65% during hibernation.

The results were eventually published with Bernie as co-author.[5,6] These became his third and fifth publications (see the chronology for the list of relevant publications).

In addition, during this time Bernie also began to experiment with a vital stain known as alizarin red S to measure bone and dental growth.[7] Clinically, he became involved with the effects of congenital syphilis on teeth[8,9] and as the war was approaching, he became engaged with the war industry work, in particular, occupational disease.[10] At the request of Dr. Schour, they wrote two war-related research papers on occupational diseases that were also eventually published.[11,12]

On reflection, the most important part of his three years at the dental school was his relationship with Dr. Isaac Schour. He was an ideal role model and mentor: his values, his ethics, his scholarship, and his philosophy were what Bernie tried to emulate for the remainder of his research career. He would spend all his free time in the research laboratory, which sometimes meant 24 hours a day. Bernie particularly treasured Saturday afternoons when he and Dr. Schour would be the only ones in the laboratory, where they would organize and write up the research material. This research regarding bones and teeth represented Bernie's early introduction to craniofacial biology. After three very busy years, Bernie received his M.S. in histology in June of 1940 and his D.D.S in August of the same year.

Military Service

In 1938, Bernie joined the Army Medical Reserve Corps and obtained a commission with the rank of first lieutenant. Later in 1939, he went for two weeks of active duty, with Fred Herzberg (a captain) and Phillip Shaneding (also a first lieutenant), to what turned out to be basic military training at Camp Custer, Michigan. Those were an intensive two weeks for medical and dental personnel and it was at that time that Bernie realized that the country was gearing up for war. Training included a 14-mile hike for which the medical personnel, including Bernie, were not sufficiently prepared. After the first few days of this regimen, feet were sore and blistered and all the muscles ached. On reporting to the first aid station for treatment, the medical officer just laughed and said: "You're doctors, take care of yourself!" Bernie also recalled one incident where they wore gas masks and had to enter a tent where mustard gas was released to simulate a gas attack. While in the tent Bernie suddenly found himself gasping for air. He soon discovered that his 'close' friend had deliberately kinked the air hose of the mask as a prank. Bernie was now faced with the unpleasant choice of whether to pull off the mask and breathe in the gas. Fortunately, his friend released the kink in the tube and Bernie was able to breathe normally. Bernie was furious with his so-called close friend who thought of it all as a big joke.

In 1942, he was called up for active duty. However, he did not pass the physical examination due to medical problems and received a deferment. After repeatedly being called up and repeatedly getting deferments, he was offered the choice of either giving up his commission or going into the inactive reserve. He chose the latter but a year later (1943), they withdrew the commission and Bernie's service days ended.

Ship's Physician

During Bernie's dental school years, he had little free time and even less money for vacations. However, through a medical friend, Bernie was able to become a ship's physician for the Cleveland and Buffalo Steamship Company or C & B.[13] This was a weekly summer cruise that left the Navy Pier in Chicago on an early Saturday evening and after a typical farewell party (balloons, confetti, etc.) steamed north toward Mackinac Island, arriving there early the next morning. From Mackinac Island, the C & B sailed to Detroit, then on to Cleveland, Buffalo and then an excursion to Niagara Falls. From Niagara Falls, the ship returned to the Navy Pier making it a seven-day cruise. It carried 750 passengers. It was commissioned by the U.S. Navy in 1942.

During that first night sailing toward Mackinac Island, Bernie and many of the passengers were down below where there was a long bar. Behind the bar was an equally long refrigerator. Bernie was sitting at the bar having a beer with other passengers, when his name was called over the loudspeaker. He was told that one of the stokers shoveling coal into the furnace was not feeling well. Bernie went to see him, and on examination found that he was in cardiac failure, clearly in serious distress. He was so far gone that

Bernie did not think he could be saved. Nonetheless, Bernie treated him and indicated that he urgently needed a hospital. Unfortunately, Mackinac Island was still eight hours away. The stoker was then put to bed to try to keep him comfortable. Bernie went back to the bar. Soon after there was a request over the loud-speaker for a priest and Bernie surmised that the stoker had died. After personally verifying that the stoker had indeed passed away, Bernie returned to the bar. There he was bombarded with questions from some of the passengers. Bernie, however, remained non-committal, but he did notice that the bartender was making room in the back of the refrigerator behind the bar. Before long they quickly shoved something clad in white about six feet long into the refrigerator. Whether the passengers ever caught on, Bernie was not able to determine. This led to a discussion between Bernie and the Captain as to what to do with the body: Keep it in the refrigerator or toss it overboard.[14] The Captain indicated that in all his years of sailing, nothing like this had ever happened before. The Captain then radioed ahead and was told to hold the body until Mackinac Island where it would be handled.

Mackinac Island was a summer retreat for the financially well off. The Island had no automobiles: You either walked, used bicycles, or horse and buggy. Not too long after arriving at Mackinac Island, Bernie was consulted by some of the ship's passengers seeking medical care. It turned out that they had partaken of the services offered by some of the women on the Island. They were now seeking help "after the fact" so to speak. While Bernie provided what treatment he could, he marveled at how they were able to find a 'house of ill-repute' on an Island that was supposedly sedate and aristocratic, catering to the wealthy. The men turned out to be sales personnel from the Ford Motor Company who were being rewarded with a week's cruise on the C & B to the Great Lakes. Most of them were there alone without their wives, which evidently provided an excuse for them to roam freely and "have a good time".

On leaving Mackinac Island, the ship headed for Detroit and then entered the Detroit River. Once up river, the Ford Motor

Company salesmen were met by their cronies who sailed out in boats to meet the ship as she steamed along. At that point, the sales people on board started tossing fifths of scotch and bourbon into the water, which were scooped up with nets. A rather strange sight, but as Bernie aptly put it: "Boys will be boys".

Bernie signed on as Ship's Doctor charged with the responsibility of giving treatment to both passengers and crew during the one week cruises. While on board, he received no salary and was not allowed to charge the passengers. Bernie, however, had the benefits of sitting at the Captain's table for meals and was treated well. Therefore, although he did not receive any pay, he did have room and board and enjoyed the cruise which, in effect, was a vacation. Since Bernie suffered from allergies, he set his 'vacation' up toward the end of summer, generally in late August, when the effects of ragweed were most pronounced in Chicago and Bernie needed to get away. Bernie served aboard the C & B in the capacity of ship's doctor for "weekly cruises" during the three years, 1939, 1940 and 1941. Having met Rhoda in July, 1941, he invited her to join him on the C & B cruise. However, she was already obligated to drive her mother and some aunts to New England at this time so she deferred. Bernie's relationship with Rhoda will take center stage in the next chapter.

Chapter 19

MARRIAGE TO RHODA E. GERARD

It would be a serious omission not to mention Bernie's marriage partner since 1941. In fact, Bernie insists that her family is the one that has a much more interesting background and could be the source of another book. Rhoda's father's family can also be traced back to the beginning of the 19th century.

One individual who stands out was Rhoda's great grandfather Jacob Ben Isaac Gesundheit (1815–1878) who was born in Warsaw, Poland. On the death of the Grand Rabbi of Warsaw in 1870, Jacob Gesundheit was chosen to succeed him. Although he had not held a rabbinic post, he was known as a great Talmudist scholar. He had headed a yeshiva, an institution for study of the Torah and the Talmud, and had written a number of books. As his views were comparatively liberal at a time of increasing conservatism, he was forced to resign four years later.[1] His son, Benjamin Gesundheit, had eleven children; the oldest of which was Maurice. In the 1880's many of the family members moved to Brighton, England.

Rhoda's father (1872–1934) Maurice,[2] a bonafide genius, who attained a wide-ranging knowledge of not only scientific fields such as astronomy and geology but also of art, history, music, opera, literature, etc. As a young man he was about to be ordained as a rabbi but he had a change of mind and heart and turned to mathematics and engineering instead. At the age of twenty, he had earned a degree in Civil and Mechanical Engineering[3] at the University of

Birmingham, England. At twenty-one, he was an assistant Professor in Engineering at Victoria University in Liverpool before eventually coming to the U.S.

He migrated from England to the U.S. around the early 1890's. He did not come through Ellis Island, as it did not exist at the time.[4] In 1898 he opened his own industrial engineering consulting firm called Gerard, Graham and Co. Over a 23-year period,[5] he successfully negotiated contracts with various companies located in Chicago as well on the East Coast. He was eventually able to count such companies as General Electric, General Motors, Rock Island Railroad, Kaiser, Westinghouse Electric, Sulzberger and Co., etc. among his many clients.

His first marriage was to Eva Teitelbaum (1872–1912), with whom he had three children: Helen (1895–1969) born in England, Ralph (1900–1974) born in Harvey, Illinois, a suburb of Chicago, and Elsie (1903–1999) born in New York. When Eva died, Maurice turned to her best friend, Florence Barnard (1875–1963), who was born in Chicago for solace. Rhoda's mother, Florence, had been a home economics teacher before she married. She had not lacked prestigious marriage proposals, such as the president of Wahl Pen Company, but had held out until someone to her liking appeared. When Maurice came along in 1914, she was thirty-nine and she accepted Maurice's marriage proposal with alacrity.

Rhoda's father was a formidable man who wielded great influence in the family. He was brilliant in thought, dominating in character and insistent in expecting that his offspring attain perfection. He had already raised a family of three by his first wife. To please his second wife, he agreed to father another child. A year later, in 1915, Rhoda Elaine Gerard was delivered by Cesarean section in Chicago when her mother was forty years of age. Rhoda was largely raised as an only child, although she knew her three half siblings. The youngest was Elsie Gerard, twelve years Rhoda's senior, and the next oldest Ralph W. Gerard, fifteen years her senior, seemed more like an uncle than a brother. The eldest sibling Helen Gerard was twenty, already married and with a baby, making Rhoda an aunt at birth. Helen lived in Pittsburgh and Rhoda saw little of her. So by that time, Helen and Ralph had been out of the house and on their own. Rhoda's impression was that some of the siblings resented her mother and never quite made their peace with her. Rhoda did see a good deal of Ralph, as he lived in Chicago and later became full professor in neurophysiology at the University of Chicago. Rhoda was also on very good terms with her other sibling, Elsie.

Rhoda's mother, a pretty woman, was the second oldest of nine children, with only her brother, Julius, being her senior. She took an active role in helping raise the seven younger siblings particularly after her mother suddenly died of a ruptured appendix.

In 1922, when Rhoda was seven, the family moved to New York to be near Wall Street and the New York Stock Exchange as Rhoda's father had retired, although only in his middle fifties, and lived on his investments that were being managed by Benjamin Graham, his nephew, who was also Rhoda's first cousin.[6]

Travel to Europe

In 1926, Rhoda's parents decided to spend two years traveling in Europe. The question that arose was what to do about Rhoda's education, as they did not want that time to be wasted. Their answer was to send her to an exclusive boarding school in Europe while they traveled. After a thorough study of various boarding schools, they settled on the Buser Töchter Institute in Teufen, Switzerland. Rhoda was not a part of the decision making process. Had she been involved, she would have undoubtedly vetoed the idea. She had never before been away from home, not even to summer camp.

Therefore, in November 1926, at the age of eleven, Rhoda was sent to the Buser Institute near Zürich for a year, while her parents traveled leisurely around Europe. While some homesickness was to be expected, Rhoda's discomfort was multiplied by the fact that German was the language exclusively spoken. It was not an easy time for a youngster who not only did not know a "ja" from a "nein," but also had never before been separated from her parents. Moreover, Herr and Frau Buser decided that for her own good, it would be better if she did not attend any classes until she understood enough German to be able to grasp what was being said. Rhoda found herself alone, day after day, not enrolled in any classes, and with no one to relate to. She ended up being miserable, suffering quietly from homesickness and loneliness. For those first weeks, she was pretty much on her own. She would go to the upper floor of the schoolhouse where there were the "Überzimmer" or piano practice rooms. During this time of isolation, when the other students would be attending classes, these rooms were vacant and Rhoda would go up there, close the door, put her head on the piano keys and cry her heart out.

The school took girls from six to eighteen years of age from all over the world. They were divided into two groups, "die kleine" and "die alte," the young and the old ones. Making connections with her fellow students was made difficult by language problems as well as the isolation of not being initially enrolled in class. A few of the students spoke English, but German was the common language.

During this time, Rhoda's parents visited her two or three times. They would meet in Zürich, which was two hours away from the boarding school in Teufen. In spite of these tearful reunions, there was no question of her being removed from the school. Her parents counseled her that once she was into a routine and got on with the rest of the girls, things would take care of themselves. They were right! After a tearful start, Rhoda managed to learn German, began to make friends, and was given permission to join the classes at the school three weeks after her arrival. In fact, she had adjusted so well to the boarding school environment that she regretted having to leave after the one year.

There were four girls assigned to each dorm room. Rhoda still remembers the names of two of them in spite of the more than seven decades that have since passed. Her best friends were Hilda Sommer from Germany and Yolanda Frugoli from Milan, Italy. Yolanda was "eine alte" at 18 years old and Rhoda really admired her. After leaving the school, Rhoda corresponded with both of them for a short while and then lost touch. In the ensuing years, she often wondered what might have happened to them, especially during WWII when both these countries were "axis powers".

Rhoda still vividly remembers Fräulein Bosshardt, the so-called housemother. She was strict but kind. One evening Rhoda found a stray kitten wandering around the grounds and, loving animals, she smuggled it under her coat and took it up to bed with her, hiding it under the covers. Needless to say, she did not get away with it as it mewed at the most inappropriate time, when Fräulein Bosshardt happened to be in the room. She snatched the kitten away much to Rhoda's bitter disappointment.

When Bernie and Rhoda were in Europe in 1973, she took him to visit Teufen in Switzerland to see the school. Nothing had changed. No new buildings, the old familiar buildings still stood there. At the entrance of the main building, visible through the open door, was a portrait of a distinguished elderly gentleman. Rhoda immediately recognized the face and exclaimed "Herr Professor Buser!" The woman who had admitted them was amazed: "Did you know him?" she asked. He was famous as the founder of the school.[7]

For the next six months, following her departure from boarding school, around January, 1927, Rhoda lived with her parents in Nice, France, in an apartment right on the Mediterranean on the Promenade des Anglais, the famous main boulevard of Nice. This time she was enrolled in one of the local elementary schools, where the spoken language was French, which like German before, was Greek to her. In an effort to help her with French, her parents hired a tutor, Madame Widovekofsky, a French-speaking Russian woman, with whom Rhoda got along well.

All subjects at the school were, naturally, taught in French. One of the daily activities was to take dictation, in French of course, from the teacher. This teacher was very understanding and without Rhoda asking, gave her permission to copy from her neighbors, telling her that it would help her learn the language. This, it turned out, was correct, but somehow Rhoda never laid down roots in that school. She made no friends and again felt isolated.

One day, thinking nothing of it, she roller-skated down the Promenade des Anglais only to be stopped and angrily berated by a gendarme for "disturbing the peace." In 1927, no one seemed to be aware in France that there was such a thing as roller skates! Another unpleasant episode occurred when Rhoda picked up and adopted a stray dog that had been wandering in the neighborhood looking forsaken. She bought a collar and leash for him and began to walk him on a daily basis. About three days later, a very irate woman grabbed the dog, all the while shouting, in French of course, accusing Rhoda of stealing him. She tore off the collar and leash and threw them at Rhoda. Not possessing adequate language skills, Rhoda was unable to explain the circumstances.

In Nice, the opera was an ongoing part of life on a weekly basis, much like going to the movies in the United States. Rhoda prepared for these occasions by taking an afternoon nap and reading the libretto of the scheduled opera, whether it was in German, French or English.

During this period in Nice, Rhoda's father organized a reunion of his family in Vichy, France, a town made famous later as the capital of the defeated French government during World War II, but at that time well-known as a health spa. Her father had siblings, nieces and nephews all over Europe and even in South Africa. As he was the oldest of eleven siblings, there were numerous relatives, none of whom Rhoda would have ever met had it not been for the reunion. Those that had been born in Poland and Austria all subsequently perished in the Holocaust. Therefore, she was doubly grateful that she was able to get to know them, if only for so short a time. Rhoda became particularly close friends with Roma Harris (Gottlieb) of Cape Town, South Africa, her first cousin, then about 20 years old. They became fast friends and corresponded for years, meeting again only once on a trip to South Africa in 1969. Another cousin that Rhoda met was Rita Auerbach, a close friend and first cousin of Roma's, from Liverpool, England. Rita eventually became the first female member of the English Parliament.

After the two-year period abroad Rhoda and her parents returned to live in New York City. They initially moved to the Bronx where she attended elementary school. Interestingly, when they had returned to New York and she had re-enrolled in school, one of the teachers asked her to stay after school one day. Rhoda wondered what she had done wrong and expected to be scolded. Instead, she said very kindly, "Rhoda, you have an excellent vocabulary, but I don't understand why you always put your verbs at the end of sentences." Rhoda did not realize that she was habitually using German syntax rules.

The family eventually moved to Brooklyn where Rhoda attended public high school. In her junior year, her father resented her teacher's behavior toward Rhoda and decided that a change of schools was needed. An incident provoked the change of schools. Rhoda had acquired painful sunburn from a day at the beach but had insisted on attending school anyway. Instead of appreciating her conscientiousness, the teacher scolded her.

This led to a move to Manhattan (86th and West End Ave.) and enrollment in Horace Mann High School, at 120th and Amsterdam across from Columbia University. This was an extremely demanding private girl's school in Manhattan that required at least an IQ of 130 to even be considered for admission. At Horace Mann, she was only an average student among peers with IQ's in the 200's. She never really felt accepted, as many of the girls had been there since kindergarten and had developed cliques, leaving her on the outside (once again). She graduated in 1931, at the age of 16, from Horace Mann and was glad that this part of her education was over. She never worked that hard again, either at UCLA or at the University of Chicago's Graduate School of Social Welfare.

While living in Manhattan, the Eva LeGallienne Civic Repertory Theatre became an important part of family life. Her parents would take Rhoda along for a weekly treat to see Shakespearean and other classic dramas. Eva LeGallienne not only starred in many productions but acted as director and producer. Rhoda admired her greatly and later corresponded with her.

Depression Years

Rhoda's father, as many others at the time, was caught in the collapse of the stock market, having lost over $100,000, a significant sum at that time.[8] He had invested heavily in the market through his nephew, Ben Graham (Rhoda's first cousin). That financial loss, coupled with the high cost of living in New York, eventually led him to move his family to Los Angeles in 1931, which at that time was much less costly.

Being only sixteen, and tired of always being the youngest, Rhoda took a year off, before attending college, enrolling in the interim at the Hollywood Secretarial School located at Hollywood and Vine. She learned stenotypy (a type of machine shorthand), typing and various other subjects of a commercial nature.[9]

One day, as she was walking home from school, as was her custom, a car stopped — an open roadster — and the driver invited her to enter. The driver was none other than Clark Gable, then in his prime. Rhoda instantly recognized him and instinctively took to her heels as far and as fast as her feet would carry her! She later learned that he had quite an eye for teenage girls.

Rhoda applied and successfully entered UCLA at the age of seventeen in 1932 and graduated as a psychology major in 1936, preparatory to obtaining professional training in social work. Rhoda had always been interested in people and what made them tick. Had her parents' financial status allowed it, she would have opted for a career as a psychiatrist or psychologist. As it was, later she often shared in the psychotherapy of patients with a psychiatrist with whom she worked with for three years, Dr. George Saslow at the Department of Psychiatry, Washington University School of Medicine, St. Louis.

Always interested in mental health, the Sarnats established an annual prize in 1992 at the National Academy of Sciences, Institute of Medicine, Washington, DC. Rosalynn Carter, the former President's wife, was the recipient for the year 2000 (Fig. 49).

Rhoda's father died suddenly in 1934 at sixty-two years of age following a prostatectomy and a pulmonary embolus. After graduation from UCLA in 1936, Rhoda and her mother moved back to Chicago where there was family and she could continue with graduate studies at the University of Chicago. Rhoda chose the Graduate School of Social Service Administration (SSA) where she earned her Master's degree in 1939.

A Career in Social Work

Rhoda studied under a number of notable scholars in the field of social work at the University of Chicago such as Edith and Grace Abbott, Charlotte Towle and Sophonisba P. Breckenridge. She finished everything except for thesis, in 1938 and earned her M. A. in 1939 as a psychiatric (now termed clinical) social worker. In her second year of fieldwork at the Psychiatric Clinic of the Michael Reese Hospital, she began a lifelong friendship with Bernice K. Simon, a fellow student, who eventually became a Distinguished Professor at SSA.

Rhoda then started her first full-time job in 1938 as a caseworker at the Jewish Social Service Bureau (JSSB). It was considered an agency with the highest professional standards that also offered the opportunity to work with a spectrum of family problems and with all age groups. Here she met someone who was to play a pivotal role in her life. This person was her supervisor, Esther Kotin Schour. While she demanded that Rhoda perform to her highest potential and accepted nothing less, she was also a deeply caring woman. She taught, guided and encouraged Rhoda, and eventually formed a close and lasting friendship.

In 1940, in her second year at JSSB, Esther Schour assigned Rhoda to supervise graduate students from SSA. Esther taught her the necessary supervisory skills and how to handle casework loads. That same year, Rhoda was elected Chairperson of the local union, the United Office and Professional Workers of America (UOPWA).

Beginnings of Married Life

How did Bernie and Rhoda first meet? It was through their respective mentors, Isaac and Esther Schour, that Rhoda met Bernie.

Isaac Schour was Bernie's chief at the University of Illinois. Bernie at that time was completing his M.S. in Histology under Schour's supervision and the D.D.S. Esther Schour, on the other hand, was Rhoda's supervisor at the JSSB.

One day Esther Schour was driving Rhoda from the JSSB branch office on the Westside of Chicago to the main office in the downtown Loop area for a case consultation with the assistant head of the JSSB, Jenny Zetland. During a lull in the conversation in the car, Rhoda piped up with the comment that she had broken up with her boyfriend. Esther gave her a quick glance, momentarily taking her eyes off the road, and asked: "Are you interested in meeting someone else?" The answer, of course, was an unhesitant "yes," particularly as someone selected by Esther would be especially meaningful. She replied: "Let me give it some thought."

Esther talked it over with her husband, Dr. Isaac Schour. They came up with several names of graduate students, with Bernie being number one on the list. Sometime later, the Histology Department in which Bernie taught was having its annual end-of-academic-year picnic. Esther also attended and took advantage of the moment to ask Bernie if he would be interested in meeting a nice young lady. Although very busy with his studies and research, his answer was in the affirmative so Esther (having come prepared) gave him Rhoda's telephone number. He finally got around to telephoning her a year later.

Rhoda shared her dating experience with one of her case workers at the Jewish Social Service Agency. Her friend was perplexed and said that this did not add up to the Bernie Sarnat that she knew. It did not. She knew Bernard D. Sarnat but not Bernard G. Sarnat. A case of mistaken identity!

Bernie, being a resident at Cook County Hospital in Chicago and earning $25 a month, did not have either much money or time available for dating. He called Rhoda for the first time on July 28, 1941, a whole year after Esther Schour told him about her at the Histology annual picnic. Rhoda sounded like someone he would like to know but, typically, work came first. However, she indicated that she was busy that night (a date with a girl friend) but hastened to add that she would be available the next evening. They clicked at that first meeting and thence forward, day by day, she was to be an increasingly important part of his life. Of course, their intermediaries, Isaac and Esther Schour, could not have been better choices from both their points of view as Rhoda worked with and under Esther's supervision and Bernie likewise did with Isaac Schour. Each of them in their own way was devoted to their respective mentors so a suggestion coming from either of them was always given serious consideration. As Bernie had little money they spent most of their time walking, talking, and taking in an occasional movie for which he had free passes (from a grateful patient) as an extra treat. Of course, Rhoda was the "rich one" then as she earned $137 per month.

She would invite him up to her apartment for refreshments. The first time Rhoda asked him to wait in the living room while she prepared the refreshments. When she did not reappear for some time, Bernie wandered into the kitchen to see what was holding things up and found her carefully reading the directions on the cocoa can. Masterfully he said, "Let me help," and in no time, there was nice, hot cocoa. Bernie, having been a Boy Scout and clerk in his father's drugstore, was a first rate fast foods cook, while Rhoda, who lived with her mother, did not do any of the cooking. Instead her talents lay in doing the dishes and cleaning up. Thus, they got to know one another and the more they knew, the more they liked what they saw.

During that period around late July or early August, 1941, Bernie had started dating Rhoda. One Sunday she came over to the hospital and was in his living quarters that he shared with Ralph Dorne, when quite unexpectedly, Bernie's mother and brother showed up. They had no idea that he was dating Rhoda. Bernie's brother Jack had just gotten married that July at the age of thirty-nine. So when Bernie's mother saw a girl sitting on his bed she wondered what Bernie was up to. Nevertheless, Rhoda was quickly accepted by Bernie's family and within four months, on Thanksgiving Day, Bernie and Rhoda were officially engaged, Bernie having finished his residency program several weeks before.

The knot was tied at the Windermere East Hotel in Chicago with Phil Shanedling as best man and Bernice Kern Simon as the matron of honor, exactly 19 days after Pearl Harbor, on Christmas Day, 1941 (Fig. 14).

However, things did not go smoothly at the wedding as Phil, the best man, who also carried the ring, was locked in the drug-store while making a telephone call after the store had closed, it being Christmas Day. Bernie, being ever resourceful, scouted down the manager who eventually released Phil so that the wedding could proceed, albeit a bit behind schedule.

The honeymoon took place in New Orleans at an uncle's house, at the Edgewater Beach Gulf Hotel in Biloxi, Mississippi and other places south (Fig. 15). As they drove down, they stayed the first night in Kankakee, Illinois, only to discover that they had to go to bed hungry, as they could not even get a cup of coffee on Christmas night, all dining places having closed. Rhoda, of course, was so excited at the noon wedding that she had eaten practically nothing. As they continued to drive south in Bernie's 1938 Plymouth, the motor overheated due to a leaking radiator. So in a little Mississippi town on a Sunday a young black boy offered to help. He took a bar of soap and plugged up the leaking radiator so that they could make it to New Orleans. Bernie and Rhoda were very grateful.

On the return from their honeymoon, in the beginning of 1942, Bernie moved in with Rhoda and her mother as the housing market was very tight at that time, in addition to the fact that neither was in a position to afford much. Bernie shared Rhoda's bedroom, which was across the hall from Rhoda's mother. While Rhoda's mother was very discreet, the same could not be said for Rhoda's cat, Pepe. Pepe was used to sleeping at the foot of Rhoda's bed (when she was single); and also having the bedroom door open. After Bernie arrived, the door was closed. In the middle of the night Pepe would mew and scratch at the closed door until let out and soon thereafter scratch and mew at the door to be let in again. This continued night after night, but Bernie was a good sport about it. This cozy "menage a quatre" ended in 1943 as Rhoda and Bernie moved to St. Louis.

It needs to be mentioned that during the war years in Chicago, Rhoda worked for the American Red Cross (ARC) as a clinical social worker, also supervising other workers. The ARC helped enlisted men and women and their families with all the problems related to their involvement in fighting World War II.

During this time Rhoda also donated blood at the American Red Cross. Once, while the blood was being drawn Rhoda fainted. The next thing she knew a doctor was slapping her face and asking her name. She replied by saying Rhoda Sarnat. He asked her if she was married and she said yes to Bernie Sarnat. He was amazed and said: "I didn't know that he was married!" That doctor and Bernie had been close friends during pre-medical and medical school at the University of Chicago. At the beginning of the war they had gone their separate ways, including marriage.

When Bernie accepted the two-year appointment in St. Louis with Dr. Blair, this meant moving there. This was a highly coveted training position as the plastic and reconstructive surgery group at St. Louis was number one worldwide at that time.

Bernie and Rhoda, with Pepe, Rhoda's cat, popped into the car, headed "south" for St. Louis. When they arrived, they were invited to stay at a large home of one of the office's secretaries until they had found a place of their own. Rhoda was initially quite worried about whether Pepe would be welcome at that home. It turned out that the secretary was also a cat lover and Pepe was greeted warmly. There were other guests there too, patients from out of town, and newcomers like Bernie and Rhoda, who could not find other accommodations. Over breakfast, they would wonder aloud about what they thought was a cat that burrowed under their covers. Yes, it was Pepe roaming, taking advantage of open doors. However, no one seemed to object so all went well. Eventually, Bernie and Rhoda were able to rent a nice apartment, where cats were welcomed, while within walking distance of the hospital.

Bernie now started as an assistant for two years in plastic and reconstructive surgery under Dr. Vilray P. Blair, a leading plastic surgeon with an international reputation and Dr. Louis T. Byars. Bernie was appointed to the surgery staff at Washington University

School of Medicine and Barnes Hospital. During his second year, Bernie was asked to stay on for an additional year (Chapter 20). Bernie worked long hours learning major reconstructive and aesthetic surgery, honing his craft.

At this time Rhoda was able to secure a position as psychiatric caseworker at the Psychiatry Clinic of the Barnes Hospital, Washington University School of Medicine. Here, in conjunction with the medical staff, she did psychotherapy with patients and supervised graduate social work students from the George Warren Brown School of Social Work at Washington University. She also supervised medical students and psychiatric residents, one of whom was Louis Gottschalk, M.D., who subsequently became Head of the Department of Psychiatry at the University of California at Irvine. It was a time of growth and learning for both Bernie and Rhoda in their respective professions. During this time at St. Louis, Gerard, their first child was born on September 13, 1945.

This brings us to early 1946 when Bernie, Rhoda and Gerry moved back to Chicago. Housing was still impossible to find as all building had been suspended during the war. Bernie's folks were generous and kind enough to take the three Sarnats in until they managed to find a place of their own. By mutual agreement, the second bedroom was given over to baby Gerry, while parents, Bernie and Rhoda, slept on a fold-out couch in the living room. A curtain hung over a rod provided what privacy there was. Both Bernie's father and mother doted on their grandson. His grandma Sarnat spent hours playing with him, while Bernie's father tended his drugstore.

After returning to Chicago, Bernie opened his first private practice office for plastic surgery on South Michigan Boulevard. He also joined the faculty of the Dental, Medical and Graduate Schools of the University of Illinois as professor and head of the Department of Oral and Plastic Surgery, where his teacher, mentor and friend, Dr. Isaac Schour, already taught. This set up a pattern of combining private practice with academia and research, which would continue into the future.

On May, 10th, 1948 along came the fourth member of the family, Joan. This completed the family, with a boy and a girl, as Bernie and Rhoda had no further plans to increase the family size. During 1951–1954 Rhoda worked as a clinical social worker and assistant district supervisor for the United Charities in Chicago.

From Chicago to Beverly Hills

Eventually Bernie and Rhoda rented their own apartment in South Shore and stayed there until 1955, when by mutual agreement, the four Sarnats moved to Beverly Hills, California.

From 1958 to 1961 Rhoda conducted a private practice in social work therapy under the auspices of the Los Angeles Psychological Service Center. It was here that a memorable incident occurred.

One day an eighteen-year-old young woman saw the sign in the window as she happened to wander by and badly in the need of help, came in. Rhoda happened to be taking applications as the intake supervisor that day and realized that this young woman was seriously mentally ill, specifically showing signs of schizophrenia. The woman insisted that she be taken on for therapy and Rhoda decided to take her on herself, which resulted in a type of "therapy," which Rhoda had never experienced before. This woman would wander aimlessly around the neighborhood for hours on end, far from where her parents lived, with Rhoda driving up one street after the other looking for her. When located, she would recognize Rhoda and without hesitation get into the car. On many an occasion, Rhoda would bring her to her own home, settle her in the "maid's room" off the kitchen, tuck her in for a night's sleep and hope for the best. This eventually culminated with Rhoda having to institutionalize her in a state psychiatric hospital where she would stay for three months or so. Rhoda visited her weekly even though this facility was a couple of hours drive away. A pattern was soon established in which she would grow increasingly disturbed upon being discharged and would need re-hospitalization about every three months.

The long-term outcome of this young woman's life is hard to believe as she eventually overcame her illness, married, had a child and, to this day, some 40 years later lives a remarkably good life with no traces of her earlier illness. The marriage has endured over all these decades and she and her husband travel, living a good life now. Rhoda still keeps in touch with her as friends. What caused this remarkable remission is unclear to this day but Rhoda is very grateful that it occurred.

In 1961, with both children in school full time, Rhoda was invited to become a faculty member of the USC Graduate School of Social Work. She started as an advisor to the graduate students in the Masters Program and subsequently became the Director of Field Work. It was a demanding but very rewarding job. This involved supervision of 125 Council agencies in several counties through a team of field instructors who she trained through her annual seminar on supervision (Fig. 42). These agencies included family and child welfare, medical psychiatry clinics and in-patient and community resources of all sorts. She worked closely with Dean Hamovitch, who was an excellent source of knowledge and support. She retired reluctantly in 1981 due to an increasingly serious hearing impairment (Fig. 45).

Esther Schour, who was still living in Chicago, suffered a serious bout of depression in 1970. Her daughter, Gabrielle, a busy psychoanalyst herself, asked her mother who she would like to have to look after her for a short period while she went on vacation. Esther, after a bit of thought said "Rhoda." So Gabrielle called Rhoda in California and Rhoda immediately offered to come and spend some time with Esther. She traveled to Chicago and spent a few weeks with her, just the two of them. It was a most meaningful experience for Rhoda to be in the position of being able to pay back some of the many kindnesses that Esther had displayed towards her over the years, even if it meant eating tuna fish (a favorite food for Esther) for both lunch and dinner throughout the period.

Retiring from USC-SSW, Rhoda decided to heed her lifelong love of animals and became a docent at the Los Angeles Zoo from about 1982 to 1993. This involved a training program which added immeasurably to her knowledge of animals. As a docent, she would escort classes of children around the zoo and lecture about animals, their lives and habits and try to answer their questions. This went on for eleven years, when, due to her deteriorating hearing, she found it increasingly difficult to understand their questions and reluctantly retired as docent as well. One of the chief benefits of this experience was meeting and becoming close friends with another docent, Barbara Gobus. This friendship has survived, despite the Gobuses moving to Southern Illinois. Thanks to the wonder of e-mail communication.

Rhoda who had developed some 70 slide shows of her various trips (see Chapter 26) then began to give talks before school children and senior citizens as well as Jewish Family Services, Jewish Community Centers and particularly at Opica, a West Los Angeles day care center for the elderly. She continued to do this until about 2003.

Part II

A CAREER IN MEDICINE
AND RESEARCH

Chapter 20

TRAINING IN PLASTIC AND RECONSTRUCTIVE SURGERY (1940–1946)

In the years 1940–41, after Bernie had finished Dental School at the University of Illinois, he decided to continue his education by taking a year's residency at the Cook County Hospital, Chicago, in Oral and Plastic Surgery. It should be mentioned that in 1939 Bernie had first applied to the Oral and Plastic Surgery, Laryngology Service at the Mayo Clinic, in Minnesota, but was not accepted.

Actually, each dental school, Loyola, Northwestern and Illinois, took one graduate into their residency program per year, usually a dentist. Bernie became the first in that residency program from the University of Illinois, Chicago at the beginning of September, 1940. He became the junior "partner" of the other two residents there.

Residency in Oral and Plastic Surgery

Bernie had been an intern at the Los Angeles County Hospital earlier and had spent time in the admitting room to see the type of patients brought in. Bernie had taken care of a number of patients with oral problems in both the Oral Surgery and the ENT[1] Combined Services at Los Angeles County Hospital. Examples of those cases included oral problems such as fractures of the jaw, lacerations, cleft lip and palate, some tumors, etc. Compared with LA County, Cook County Hospital, Chicago, was more diverse and extensive in variety of its intake of patients. That is, the patient load and the pathologies they exhibited were considerably more varied and advanced.

For the first four months Bernie was the third resident in line. He was really there to learn and to assist the two senior residents. But the residents would let him do certain procedures. Then, later as senior resident, Bernie took the more difficult cases. At Cook County Hospital, there were a tremendous number of fractures of the jaws and fractures of the zygoma or cheek bones. As one of the three residents, he would treat most of the patients on an out-patient basis. However, hospital beds were available to treat the more serious cases.

Bernie recalled with affection the various members (attendees) of the staff who oversaw the residents. In particular, there was William H. G. Logan, M.D., D.D.S., who was at that time Dean of the Loyola School of Dentistry (formerly the Chicago College of Dentistry). Dr. Logan was the son-in-law of Dr. Truman W. Brophy, a very famous oral/plastic surgeon who had an international repu-tation in the repair of cleft lip and palate. Dr. Logan, in some ways, was following in his father-in-law's footsteps. Dr. Logan had also been in charge of oral and dental surgery during World War I. Clearly, he was an outstanding individual. However, it should be noted that by the time Bernie started as a resident, Logan was semi-retired and would only be seen infrequently. As a consequence, Dr. Logan was rarely involved in the day-to-day surgical activities.

The other attendee was Joseph Schaefer, who also had an M.D., D.D.S. like Logan, but with a law degree as well and was some-thing of an artist. Under his supervision surgeries were not limited to oral and maxillofacial surgery, but included rhinoplasty,[2] flaps, skin grafts for burns and other procedures. Dr. Schaefer was inspir-ing, colorful, if somewhat eccentric; nevertheless, he was a good teacher and Bernie learned much from him.

So during the course of this year, Bernie saw a wide variety of problems including tumors of the neck, face, jaws and mouth, all sorts of trauma, fractures, lacerations, diseases of the mouth and face. Bernie recalled that as a senior resident he was operating on a patient with a thyroglossal duct cyst on an outpatient basis. One has to remember that this was 1940, well before outpatient surgery become popular, starting in the 1960's.

Bernie would be on call every third night. Being on call entailed a 24-hour vigil at the hospital. In particular, Friday and Saturday nights were especially busy nights for the surgical service. Cases such as shotgun and stab wounds would come in and have to be treated. While many of the cases would be first seen in the emergency room, later they would be sent to the specific service involved in the treatment. He made good friends while in the residency program. In fact, one of them at that time, Ralph Dorne, his roommate, a resident in ENT in Santa Monica, California. Bernie has maintained this relationship since 1940. Dorne retired from practice in 2007.

His routine as resident included making rounds in the morning seeing patients in the hospital before beginning the surgical schedule of inpatients suffering from such varied ailments as gunshot wounds, burns, skin grafts, etc. Also involved would be cases with cleft lip/palate that had been operated on. By 1:00-1:30 pm, he would be in the outpatient clinic seeing 30–40 patients in an afternoon. This entailed checking the course of treatment of old patients and following the admittance of new patients, as well as different seminars and teaching conferences. With his residency nearly completed, he was asked by Dr. Logan if he would teach some of the biology courses. So, in September, 1941, Bernie then took a position at Loyola University Dental School and taught for the next academic year.

At this time, he had become aware of the newly formed Board in Plastic Surgery that required two years of general surgery and two years of training in general plastic surgery. So he came home one day and indicated to Rhoda (they had been married for less than two months) that this was what he wanted to do next. Rhoda, without any hesitation said "go for it."

Assistantship in General Surgery

Bernie applied for general surgical training under Dr. Marshall Davison at University Hospital, Chicago and he was accepted as a junior assistant starting in September, 1942. This was after Bernie and Rhoda had spent the worst of the hay fever and asthma season in the upper peninsula of Michigan. Bernie's longstanding problems with hay fever will eventually play a major part in his move to California.

University Hospital was practically across the street from Cook County Hospital. Marshall Davison's father Charles Davison, an outstanding surgeon in his own right, was the founder of University Hospital. Interestingly, Marshall Davison had evidently read Bernie's work on alizarin red S[3] as he indicated that his father also had done research with dogs using alizarin red S a generation earlier. Bernie thinks Davison's work was on long bones but it has remained unpublished. For Bernie, Marshall Davison was a wonderful role model.

Bernie, as the junior resident to Dr. Davison, was exposed to general surgery. In his year there, Bernie did herniotomies, hemorrhoidectomies, appendectomies, tonsillectomies, adenoidectomies, and a few cholecystectomies. In addition, of course, he assisted on a wide variety of other surgical procedures. All in all, it was a good learning experience in general surgery.

While normally two years of general surgical training was required, Bernie also learned that the American Board of Plastic Surgery was willing to accept a year of research in lieu of the second year of general surgery. Since Bernie had obtained a masters degree in research and published a certain number of scientific papers by that time, the Board required him to complete only one year of general surgery.

Now Bernie needed to get plastic surgery training. With Rhoda's help, they sent letters to a number of different plastic surgeons hoping that one of them might have a training program. There were no formal residencies. The only one was at the Mayo Clinic, and that program was not accepted by the Board because it was limited to surgery above the clavicles. The Board insisted that the whole body be involved in the training of plastic surgeons.

So Bernie wrote letters to various outstanding plastic surgeons such as Staige Davis at Johns Hopkins, to Vilray Blair in St. Louis, to Ferris Smith in Grand Rapids and Kazanjian in Boston who was originally a dentist but obtained an M.D. later at Harvard. Bernie heard back from Kazanjian, who indicated that he had his nephew with him so there was no opening. Davis also wrote back indicating there was nothing available in his department. Bernie never heard from either Smith or Blair.

Assistantship in General Plastic and Reconstructive Surgery

In January 1943, Bernie received a letter from Marshall Davison inviting him to a luncheon at the Chicago Athletic Club at which some outstanding physicians such as Sumner Koch, Mike Mason, and the Chair of the Department of both Surgery and Neurosurgery at Northwestern, Loyal Davis (father-in-law to Ronald Reagan), were present. Much to Bernie's surprise, Vilray Blair was also present and wanted to meet him. Bernie, being just a resident at that time, was quite awed by the presence of so many internationally known and distinguished surgeons. After the luncheon, Bernie was able to have a talk with Dr. Blair, who offered him a contract, for two years with a salary of $200 a month if he would come to St. Louis. Bernie was ecstatic at the opportunity! The famous Dr. Blair, who had been head of the section of maxillofacial and plastic surgery in the United States Army and chief consultant in maxillofacial surgery with the American Expeditionary Forces during World War I, had now accepted Bernie to be his first assistant for two years and even with salary. Bernie felt privileged to be able to learn from one of the giants in plastic surgery.

While Bernie planned to finish his general surgical training under Davison until the end of August 1943, Blair asked Davison if he could release Bernie a bit earlier as they were in urgent need of help in St. Louis. So Bernie and Rhoda left Chicago in May,

1943 and started work under the capable leadership of Vilray P. Blair and Louis T. Byars, both world famous plastic surgeons at Barnes Hospital, Washington University Medical School, St. Louis. Rhoda and Bernie were greeted most warmly soon after they arrived for a Sunday afternoon tea at Dr. Blair's home, where they met his wife and members of the family.

Dr. Blair was devastated when Kathryn, his wife, suffered a severe stroke and hemiplegia. So that she would not be house-bound, he had a large bus converted into a mobile home-hospital. Because the brothers (and family) who at that time controlled General Motors were patients of his, they cooperated fully in constructing the bus to Dr. Blair's detailed specifications. The bus included an elevator so that the wheelchair could be rolled out at street level. At least five people could sleep onboard. There was a complete kitchen with cooking stoves and refrigerator, a bathroom, air-conditioning, etc. A full-time chauffeur, Blair's handyman, could also be accommodated. Now he and his "missus" could travel as desired. He was very proud of his bus.

This was the beginning of two very busy years for Bernie. When the two years were over and Bernie was planning to return to Chicago, Dr. Blair asked him if he would consider a third year. Bernie was flattered to be asked and accepted, resulting in a very productive and rewarding three-year stay in St. Louis.

The Vilray P. Blair Group

Bernie was now to spend three of the most important and satisfying years of his life in St. Louis. The time spent in St. Louis was particularly memorable for Bernie as it allowed him to really sharpen the tools of his specialty; namely, the practice of plastic and reconstructive surgery. These three years from 1943 through 1946 were busy and filled with learning. As a full-time assistant to both Drs. Blair and Byars and a member of the private practice office staff, Bernie had received appointments to both the faculty of the

Department of Surgery at Washington University School of Medicine and Barnes Hospital.

The office of the Vilray P. Blair Group was located in the Metropolitan Building, at Grand and Olive streets in St. Louis. It was large, spacious but plainly furnished. The waiting room could seat 40 patients comfortably. There were several examining rooms and several offices for personnel. The surgical staff now included Bernie, Vilray P. Blair, Louis T. (Bill) Byars, Frank McDowell, and James B. Brown, who was in the military service at the time (Valley Forge Hospital) but returned on occasion. Two full-time registered nurses completed the professional staff.

Bernie subsequently learned that Dr. Blair had wanted his son, who was a physician, to join the office staff. Dr. Brown had blocked this appointment, hurting Blair immeasurably. So the son, instead, became an orthopedic surgeon. Bernie also learned that there were two separate and independent administrative staffs. He was certainly not aware that there was a schism in the office and never did learn the cause of it. Della O. Cooper was the financial secretary exclusively working for Drs. Blair and Byars, while Mr. Hance worked exclusively for Drs. Brown and McDowell. Miss Fahrni was Dr. Blair's full-time secretary, and Estelle Hillerich was part-time office and part-time American Board of Plastic Surgery secretary. Gertrude Hance (sister of Mr. Hance) was the full-time photographer, artist, tattooist, and prosthetist. A handyman ran errands and performed other services. Office hours usually began at about 2.00 pm (following a morning of surgery) and sometimes lasted until 6.00 or 7.00 pm. During the busy summer the staff would see as many as 100 patients per day, who came from near and far. Some had very complex problems and Blair and Byars enjoyed the challenge. Every socioeconomic class and age group was represented. No one was ever turned away.

Dr. Blair, then 72 years old, was by then performing surgery only three days a week. In the afternoon, Bernie and Miss Fahrni would accompany him to see new patients. He would dictate the history and examination and his plan for the surgical procedure the next day. Bernie would then bring that information to surgery.

Frequently, partway through the operation, Bernie would be lost. Blair with his nimble hands and brilliant mind had thought of a new and better approach. Bernie became responsible for the post-operative care of all of Dr. Blair's and some of Dr. Byars' patients.

One afternoon, Dr. Blair asked him to answer a letter from a general practitioner in western Missouri who could not be certain of the sex of his five-year-old patient. Bernie thought that by that time he was quite knowledgeable and arranged for the child's visit. After examining the patient, he too was bewildered. Briefly, there were what appeared to be labia majora in which he could palpate small round masses, which proved to be rudimentary testicles. There was a partially developed introitus and what appeared to be a rather large clitoris. After Dr. Blair examined the patient, he also could not decide the sex of this child, who had been raised and dressed as a girl and who clutched a doll. Blair decided to do an abdominal exploratory procedure. He found a rudimentary uterus and ovaries, leading to his decision that the child continued to be raised as a girl. This was 1944.

Della O. Cooper managed the office for Dr. Blair until 1950 and was in charge of making appointments. After Dr. Blair had seen a new patient, she set the surgical fees and arranged for hospital admission, temporary housing and other matters. In addition, Cooper conducted a rather active business in the delivery of radium needles and radon gold seeds to various outside medical consumers. At one time Dr. Eliis Fischel, a prominent head and neck surgeon and radiation oncologist, had his office with Dr. Blair. Blair apparently inherited his radiation company, which eventually was turned over to Della Cooper.

After the very busy summer practice slowed down, particularly during the winter, the staff turned to other medical matters. One day Dr. Blair called in Miss Fahrni and asked her to gather the last 100 records of patients with partial and total nasal reconstructions with pedicle flaps. Bernie assisted Dr. Blair over many afternoons in reviewing and organizing this material for publication. Dr. Blair eventually submitted the manuscript to Dr. Loyal Davis, then editor of Surgery, Gynecology, and Obstetrics. Bernie overheard a telephone call from Dr. Davis asking Dr. Blair for a title other than, "Hits, Strikes, and Outs." Blair was adamant and his title remained intact.[4]

This was without question the finest plastic surgery training program at that time. Yet, even by 1947, there were only nine formal residency programs in plastic surgery. Needless to say, the more than 100 present-day plastic and reconstructive surgery residency programs are far superior in both breadth and depth.[5]

Several excellent reports give many details of the life of Vilray P. Blair (1871–1955).[6] The following comments are limited to how Bernie remembered him, principally in the years he was his first assistant, from 1943 through 1946. He was a fairly tall (certainly when compared to Bernie), rather stooped, formidable-appearing gentleman with a shock of gray hair. Although he was soft-spoken, his voice was commanding. He was a man of the utmost integrity.

Blair would often telephone Bernie at home at unusual hours. Sometimes he would inquire about the postoperative condition of a patient. Other times, at 6.00 am, Bernie would join him for a visit to a convent, where Blair gave general medical care to the nuns, and from there they would go to Mass, which Blair attended every morning before surgery. Some trips were to a special horse farm, where Blair would carefully inspect the tails, looking for the optimum horsehair for surgical sutures. From time to time they would travel to the Veterans Administration Hospital at Jefferson Barracks, near St. Louis, to do surgery. On rare occasions, they would perform surgery at other hospitals.

The American Association of Oral Surgeons, a forerunner of the American Board of Plastic Surgery, was formed in 1923 by three double-degreed (M.D., D.D.S.) men in Chicago, representing the heads of the oral and plastic surgery departments in the three dental schools (Brophy-Chicago College of Dental Surgery, Gilmer-Northwestern University Dental School, and Moorehead-University of Illinois College of Dentistry). For several years, those with a general surgical background, but without a dental degree, were not admitted. These included Vilray Blair, John Staige Davis, Ferris Smith and others. The rules were later changed, and they were finally admitted.

Blair was the driving force that established the Board. His concept was that a plastic surgeon should have at least two years of general surgical experience before going into the specialty. A second concept was to bring the various plastic surgery subspecialties under one umbrella (oral surgery, otolaryngology, ophthalmology, head and neck surgery, hand surgery, genitourinary surgery, aesthetic surgery, etc.)

Blair traveled the country in the 1930's and would hold dinner meetings to assess the status of plastic surgery in the United States. Once he related to Bernie his visit in 1937 to Los Angeles. In talking with Arthur Smith, M.D., D.D.S., they discussed temporomandibular joint surgery and the hockey stick incision. Blair asked about the scar, and Smith reputedly said that he never left a scar.

Otto Bames, William Kiskadden and Emil Tholen were admitted to the board. Not accepted were Balsinger, Felsen, Gaynor, McGee, Smith (he sued the board unsuccessfully), and Updegraff. In Chicago, Sumner Koch, W. H. G. Logan, Michael Mason, Fred Merrifield, Frederick Moorehead, and Louis Schultz, Sr., were grandfathered in. Again, not included were Samuel Salinger, Joseph Schaeffer, Louis Schultz, Jr., and Max Thorek.

When it came time to elect the first officers of the newly formed American Board of Plastic Surgery, Blair was the unanimous choice for president. However, he deferred, saying that he would be more effective as secretary. He instead championed John Staige Davis as president.

As mentioned earlier, Dr. James B. Brown (1899–1971) joined Dr. Blair's practice in 1925. Brown had been in the military service during most of the period of 1943–1946, first in the European Theater and then at Valley Forge Hospital in Pennsylvania. Brown would return periodically, more often by 1946. Although Bernie had met him on several occasions, he felt that he knew him the least well of those in the group. Famous surgeons who trained under Brown were Bradford Cannon, Joseph Murray, Peter Randall, Erle Peacock, Ralph Millard, Josh Jurkiewicz, and Carl Hartrampf.[6] Brown died as a result of hypertension and a stroke.

Dr. Louis T. (Bill) Byars (1906–1969) joined the Blair group in 1935 and Bernie spent much close time with him. He was a quiet, somewhat shy, undemonstrative, unusually fine, modest, extremely capable, and gentle but firm man. Bill Byars was undoubtedly one of the most consummate and masterful surgeons that Bernie had the fortune to know. From 1943 through 1946, he carried the workload of the group, operating six days a week. His varied surgical capabilities were most remarkable, and not once did Bernie observe a surgical failure. Although he had received national recognition, Bernie doubted that Dr. Byars was ever as fully appreciated as he deserved.

Bernie and Bill Byars produced several publications[7–10] together and he wrote the foreword to a book that Bernie had co-authored.[11] Periodically, Dr. Byars invited Rhoda and Bernie to his home for Saturday night dinner. He treasured those evenings. With a Scotch and soda in hand, they would sit around a crackling fire and leisurely review the past week's doings at the office and hospital and the state of the specialty of plastic surgery in general. Bill had married "Bam" in 1936. Bam was a wonderful, gracious hostess who made everyone feel at ease and, interestingly, was the sister of Dr. Brown's first wife. Their daughter, Caroline, a pretty child, was born in 1939. It was Bill Byars (with an assist from Brad Cannon) who encouraged Robin Anderson and Milt Edgerton to organize the Plastic Surgery Research Council, of which Bernie was a founding member in 1955 and chairperson in 1957. When Bernie developed a Dukes' C carcinoma of the bowel in 1961, it was Bill Byars who gave him much needed counseling. Tragically, Byars died of a carcinoma of the prostate.

Dr. Frank McDowell (1911–1981) joined the group in 1939. Frank was a true scholar, quiet, reserved, and somewhat withdrawn. From 1943 through 1946, he carried on the surgical practice of Dr. Brown and did considerable writing with him. Although Bernie had a cordial relationship with him, he did not work as closely with Frank as he did with Drs. Blair and Byars. He did scrub with him at times if he had an interesting or difficult surgical problem. One time, while he was scrubbing, a child while being given anesthesia by a nurse anesthetist suddenly died. Frank broke his scrub, ran into the operating room, and practically went berserk. He later moved to Hawaii to practice; under his editorship, Plastic and Reconstructive Surgery became an outstanding and significant journal. Sadly, he died of a carcinoma of the bowel.

Bernie's Years with the Vilray Blair Group

Fortunately, at the same time that Bernie was a member of the Vilray P. Blair Group, Rhoda had received an appointment in the Department of Psychiatry as a psychiatric social worker assisting and working with Drs. Gildea and Saslow. This proved to be a most valuable learning experience for her. Sometimes some of the plastic surgery patients would be shared with the Department of Psychiatry and conversely.

Bernie began organizing his 25 case reports for the American Board of Plastic Surgery during June and July of 1945. These cases were later used to document Bernie's skills in Plastic Surgery as part of the requirements for Board certification (Chapter 22).

At that time, Rhoda was six months pregnant. They would go to the record room at Barnes Hospital on Sunday mornings, and she would help him transcribe the necessary records of patients with all manner of deformities. They wondered, although they never shared their thoughts, would their child be born with a deformity? They were most fortunate in eventually having a healthy, vigorous baby boy who later went on to Harvard College and eventually to the Stanford Medical School.

In addition to his responsibilities as assistant to Drs. Blair and Byars, Bernie was also appointed as plastic surgeon-in-charge at Homer Phillips and St. Louis City Charity Hospitals. Dr. H.B.G. Robinson, professor and head of Oral Pathology at Washington University School of Dentistry became a good friend, and invited Bernie to give several lectures. When Robinson left for Ohio State University School of Dentistry, Dr. Barnet Levy succeeded him, and he also became a very close colleague and personal friend of Bernie. In lecturing to his classes, he became acquainted with several of his students (George Bernard, Marvin Burstone and Robert Gorlin) who subsequently became well-known in their fields.

In 1945, Dr. LeRoy Main, a dental radiologist and Dean of St. Louis University Dental School, a long-time friend of Dr. Blair's, invited Bernie to become full professor and head of the Department of Oral and Plastic Surgery. Bernie was indeed highly flattered and, of course, very pleased. He stated that he was definitely interested but with several provisos: (1) he would need Dr. Blair's permission to take on this added responsibility, (2) he would probably require approval from Washington University to be on the staff of another university faculty, and (3) he eventually planned to return to Chicago. Dr. Blair and Chancellor Compton gave immediate approval, and Dr. Main was not concerned about his probable return to Chicago. So Bernie added further challenges to an already very full program. At the St. Louis University School of Dentistry, Bernie met William Bauer, M.D., D.D.S, an outstanding oral pathologist who was professor and head of the department.

As Bernie was completing his program, he informed Dr. Blair about his plans to leave St. Louis. By this time Bernie had developed enough of a private practice that he was earning income far beyond his office salary. As time approached to depart, Bernie mentioned that he might be interested in moving to Los Angeles. Blair communicated this to Dr. Kiskadden, a great devotee of Dr. Blair's, in Los Angeles. He was, however, quite discouraging, saying that there were already too many plastic surgeons in Los Angeles. So, the three Sarnats decided to move back to Chicago in 1946. Bernie would return to St Louis for a few days each month to honor his commitment to the St. Louis University School of Dentistry. Later in 1946, he was offered (not unexpectedly) and accepted a professorship as head of the Department of Oral and Plastic Surgery at the University of Illinois College Of Dentistry in Chicago as it was known then. This position had been previously held by Dr. Frederick B. Moorehead, one of the three founding members of the American Association of Oral Surgeons — the future American Association of Plastic Surgeons. Bernie became a diplomate of the American Board of Plastic Surgery in 1947.

He also joined Paul Greeley[12] in the Division of Plastic Surgery of he College of Medicine at the University of Illinois.

In 1949 Blair invited Bernie to join him in St. Louis where he received an honorary degree from Washington University. In December 1955, the very week that Vilray P. Blair died, the four Sarnats moved permanently from Chicago to Los Angeles. Thus, Bernie regretfully relinquished a full professorship, head of department, tenure, a pension, a very active graduate program, and a 10-year private practice of plastic surgery to start anew in Los Angeles. It is with gratitude that he is listed as the last one of the famous plastic surgeons who trained under Vilray P. Blair, along with Jerome Webster, Earl Padgett, J. B. Brown, Louis Byars, Frank McDowell, William Hamm, and Minot Fryer.[6]

Barnes Hospital

Practically all surgical procedures were performed at Barnes Hospital, although from time to time they worked at nearby Jewish Hospital. At Barnes there were two adjoining surgical suites. Blair and Byars used the larger one, which housed two operating tables. The other suite with one operating table was used by McDowell and Brown. In the major suite, all walls and the ceiling had been decorated with paintings from nursery rhymes — Jack Horner, Little Miss Muffett, Jack and the Beanstalk, Tommy Tucker, etc. With this as an addition, Bernie often wondered what emotions the patients experienced under the influences of the preoperative medication and their fears. Visiting surgeons were always intrigued. The surgical nurse, Miss McDavitt, would scrub up at about 8.00 am and gather all of the sterile surgical equipment and dressings for the day on her central table. She would stay scrubbed and sterile all day (Bernie never saw her go to the bathroom) and would supply the two surgeons with the necessary surgical materials. Thus, there was less delay between surgical procedures.

Blair would use a gauze mask and wear his old tennis shoes. During the scrub period, Bernie found it particularly enjoyable because he would love to either hum or share his reminiscences with him. Those were especially treasured memories for Bernie.

In the early 1900's Blair would take the night train to Chicago to observe on the next day, the work of Brophy on cleft lip and palate patients. After several years, Blair was disappointed with his clinical surgical results, and by 1917, he had discarded Brophy's technique. The method required passing wires to hold the compressed maxillae together, resulting in several deformities of the maxillae and developing teeth. This led to an excellent, detailed study by Logan and Kronfeld.[12] In searching for other methods, Blair ended with using the modified Mirault and von Langenbeck procedures. He said that he deliberately did not publish his results until after Brophy had died in the 1920's. Blair also related his acquaintance with Edward Angle, the world-famous orthodontist then practicing in St. Louis in the early 1900's. Apparently Angle had a patient with a prognathic mandible, and he prevailed upon Blair to operate by extracting the bicuspids and the corresponding sections of the mandible. Blair said that the surgical result was a disaster, and after that episode he switched to the transramal cut. He would talk about his high esteem for and fondness of Robert Ivy, who worked closely with him in the U.S. Army during Work War I. Blair, invited Ivy to join him in his practice in St. Louis after the war but Ivy declined and returned to Philadelphia. However, they did coauthor a book, *The Essentials of Oral Surgery*, which was published in several editions.

The surgical schedule began at 8.30 am and continued until about 2.00 pm, when they would leave for the office. There was hardly time for lunch. In the basement of Barnes Hospital was a small lunch counter, where Bernie would take about 10 minutes off for a quick hamburger and a Coke. Frank McDowell would join him frequently but not Bill Byars. Bernie did not think that he ever ate lunch.

On Saturdays they would not go to the office, instead they operated until as late as 5.00 pm, especially in the summer. As Bernie became more experienced, he was given the responsibility for the second surgical table on days that Dr. Blair did not operate, and particularly on Saturdays, when they (using all three surgical tables) would operate on as many as 25 patients. Thus, in a single day one could see the complete gamut of plastic and reconstructive surgery: toe-to-thumb transplants, hypospadias repair, forehead flap used to reconstruct the nose, neck dissection, cleft lip, skin grafting of burns, rhinoplasty, facelift, etc.

Blair had mentioned to Bernie that in the early 1900's he even did some neurosurgery. While there, a surgical resident's wife gave birth to a child with an exstrophy of the urinary bladder. We transplanted the ureters to the large bowel and eventually closed the defect.

One patient's episode in 1944 that remains vividly in Bernie's mind was that of the actress Carmen Miranda. After several unsuccessful surgical procedures on her nose in Los Angeles, she came to see Dr. Blair in St. Louis. In her movies she was wearing a false nose to cover the deformity. Two incidents: On the first occasion, she arrived with her entourage — mother, sister, business manager, and beautician — and they occupied an entire large penthouse suite at the Park Plaza Hotel. She apparently received an appropriate bill from Della Cooper, because the next time she arrived with only her sister Aurora. During surgery on her first visit, and while under local anesthesia and the influence of the preoperative medication, which undoubtedly lessened her inhibitions, she began to sing and move her hips, and suddenly she pulled off the sheet and was completely in the nude. At that point Blair read her the riot act, which immediately subdued her behavior, and from then on she never pulled any more high jinks.

The second incident was on her return visit, after having undergone a second-stage, relatively benign procedure. That evening about 7.00 pm, the nurse at Barnes Hospital called and told Bernie that Miranda's oral temperature was 102° F. He immediately went to the hospital and found that her white blood cell count was 12,000 per mm. The surgical wound did not appear to be unusual, but there was some tenderness to palpation mostly in the right lower quadrant of the abdomen. The menstrual period did not seem to be relevant. Bernie telephoned Dr. Blair who arrived at about 8.00 pm. He had nothing to offer and telephoned Dr. Evarts Graham, Chief of Surgery. He arrived about an hour later with his staff, and they, too, were perplexed. The decision was to do an exploratory procedure through a right rectus incision. The findings were not helpful. With the beginning of closure, Nathan Womack in the gallery called out, "Biopsy the liver," which was done. Dr. Byars, the plastic surgeon, closed the skin. The postoperative course was uneventful. The biopsy report was multiple amoebic abscesses. The skin wound developed a keloid scar, which required subsequent treatment. In the meantime, back in Hollywood, her costumes, because of the scar, shielded areas usually exposed! Bernie and Rhoda did have her sister, Aurora, over to their modest apartment for dinner. She was a delightful person and had appeared in one of Disney's earliest films with Mickey Mouse.

Blair and Byars were most generous in sharing their knowledge, which was not always the case for other plastic surgeons of that time. Any ethical surgeon was always welcome to observe. Visitors came from throughout the United States and from abroad. Earlier, after a visit with Blair's group, Jerome Webster returned to Columbia University to establish his formal residency program there. Ken Pickrell, after three months of observation, initiated his residency program at Duke. Bill Longmire was on the same track but eventually chose to stay in general surgery and became chairman of the Department of Surgery at the University of California, Los Angeles. Ralph Millard also spent some time with them. Just before, during, and just after his three-year stay, the following spent variable amounts of time in the plastic surgery service at Barnes Hospital: Robin Anderson, McCarthy De Mere, Sanford Dietrich, Milton Edgerton, Merton Hatch, Gordon Letterman, Allyn McDowell, Frank Meany, Peter Randall, and Robert Robinson.

Chapter 21

LIFE IN ST. LOUIS AND CHICAGO

Housing was scarce in St. Louis as it was elsewhere during World War II. Bernie and Rhoda rented temporary living quarters with Mrs. Hillerich (one of Dr. Blair's secretaries). Mrs. Hillerich owned a stately mansion with many rooms. She would rent them out to patients of Dr. Blair's and their families who were from out of town. As they drove up they were a bit apprehensive since they had not mentioned that they had a cat. As Mrs. Hillerich opened the door, Bernie said that there were three members of the family. At which point she asked: Was it a boy or girl? Bernie replied that it was a cat. To which she responded: We love cats! The Sarnats and Pepe the cat were, of course, delighted to receive such a warm and enthusiastic welcome. After a few days they began to learn from some of the other tenants that something was crawling into their beds and tunneling under their blankets. Bernie and Rhoda tried to restrain Pepe but this was, of course, difficult. This was May 8, 1943.

By June, they are able to obtain a hotel room at the Forest Park Hotel several blocks away but near Barnes Hospital. This room was on the fifth floor facing east. In the morning, they would get the hot St. Louis sun, which was quite uncomfortable, but at least they had their own place. However, there were a few disquieting factors. On Friday and Saturday evenings, the bar across the street on the first floor would have live entertainment and libations. The bar patrons would become a bit noisy and this would last until three in the morning keeping the Sarnats up most of the night.

Another complicating factor was the need for summer doors. These doors had about eight to 10 inches open at the bottom and about eight to 10 inches open at the top to permit ventilation during the hot summers. These openings allowed access to the hallway. Pepe could not be restrained and would wander into the hallway and go into the other rooms. Next door was an old-timer who complained to the management whereupon the management gave the Sarnats 10 days notice to vacate.

Once again, Mrs. Hillary came to their rescue, as she knew of a woman who also loved cats. Bernie and Rhoda went out there and saw that she had eight or ten cats all around the house. She welcomed Pepe, he seemed to make the adjustment, and so they left him there. They would visit him at regular intervals and would find him sitting inside a large fruit bowl on the dining room table. He seemed to be very content.

Most fortunately, by September of 1943, the Sarnats were able to obtain an apartment at 4405 West Pine Street. It was a small apartment in a building where one of the office nurses (Miss Phelps) also lived. This was the exact building that they were looking for. The Ellsworth building was a relatively new modern six-story building with an elevator. It was well located near Barnes Hospital; it was quiet. In addition, the cat was welcome. In short, it was a place that they could call home, and they lived in it until they left for Chicago in February of 1946.

However, as summers were unbearably hot in St. Louis, Dr. Blair was most considerate and had an air-conditioning window unit (such as it was) installed for them. There was no bedroom. Instead, a Murphy bed was pulled down each evening in the living room. Adjoining was a walk-in closet and bathroom. When Gerry, their son, came along in September 1945, they kept him and his crib in the walk-in closet.

Living in St. Louis During the War Years

Living in St Louis during the war meant rationing. Red stamps, for example, were for protein, meats, cheese and canned fish. They had to use these stamps very carefully because of the cat that was finicky and would eat only canned fish. However, one marketing day, Bernie discovered a canned fish known as Piltchard's that did not require red stamps. One day, while in line, a woman asked if this canned fish was any good, Bernie did not have a heart to tell the woman that it was for the cat. He suspected that she used it for regular human consumption.

Other rationed items included gasoline. However, as Bernie was a physician, he did get a limited number of coupons for gasoline. Although he used them conservatively for going to the office, hospital and making rounds, he did occasionally have more than he needed. With this excess, they took a trip to the Ozark Mountains of Western Missouri for a small vacation.

When Rhoda would go to work in the morning at Barnes Hospital, she would stop by the nearby market and ask if there were any meat available. The butcher then indicated that when she came by after work he would have a little something for her. That afternoon, she would stop by and there would be a small package for her. When she came home and opened the package, it usually contained a little cube steak, barely enough for the two of them, but they were delighted to have it. Once a week, on Thursday evenings, Rhoda and Bernie would do their weekly marketing at a large supermarket known as Bettendorf's, located in western St. Louis. It was a wonderful supermarket at the time. They would also take Mrs. Hillerich and her adult daughter along as well. They would have supper in the cafeteria and then do their marketing.

Occasionally, Rhoda would be able to buy a duck. The weekly budget for groceries was about five dollars. On Sunday, Rhoda would put the duck in the Nesco, an electric oven, set the timer, and then they would take Gerry out for a Sunday afternoon ride. When they returned to the apartment it would be full of wonderful cooking aromas.

An epicurean highlight was going to Rugerri's in South St. Louis. There, one could get a most wonderful steak (tenderloin, sirloin, t-bone, filet, etc.) dinner without the use of red stamps. Bernie often wondered what their source of this generally unavailable meat was. Of course, they could not afford this wonderful dinner very often. Living in St. Louis during World War II, they were busy all week with relatively few opportunities for leisure time.

In February 1946, with Gerry now five months old, the three Sarnats jumped into their economy model Plymouth and Bernie drove Rhoda and Gerry to the airport and saw them off to Chicago. Rhoda and Gerry were met at Chicago's Midway airport by Bernie's brother Jack who took them to the apartment of Bernie's parents.

Bernie then drove the Plymouth back to their apartment, loaded up all of their belongings and headed north for the six-hour drive to Chicago. Bernie left St. Louis looking forward to his future life back in Chicago.

Returning to Chicago

Those had been very important and busy years in St. Louis from 1943 until 1946. Bernie and Rhoda were now back in Chicago and starting anew in their personal lives and careers. For Bernie this meant: (1) finding a place to live and care for his family; (2) establishing a new practice in plastic and reconstructive surgery; and (3) renewing his academic and scientific career.

When Bernie and Rhoda arrived in Chicago from St. Louis they were not able to find a place to live at first and his parents were good enough to let the three of them into their two-bedroom apartment. Bernie and Rhoda lived with his parents from February 1946 until April 1947 due to the shortage of housing. While Bernie's parents slept in one of the bedrooms, Gerry, now approaching one-year old, slept in the other bedroom, and Bernie and Rhoda slept on a couch that opened up in the living room.

It must be recalled that this was less than a year after the end of World War II and things were still shifting from a war to a peace-time economy. Bernie was grateful that they were able to stay with his parents who doted upon Gerry. His mother would often baby sit allowing Bernie and Rhoda an occasional evening out. With the family drugstore only two blocks away, Rhoda, who was now not working, would wheel Gerry in the baby buggy, especially during the winter months, to the drugstore. Bernie's father, who was very accommodating, would make a hot chocolate for Rhoda. This gave Rhoda a chance to get out a bit. Gena Weinmann, wife of Dr. Peter Weinmann who was a colleague of Bernie's, would join Rhoda with her baby daughter Cathy, and they would wheel their buggies together and converse, etc. Gena had been formerly married to the world famous psychologist Bruno Bettelheim who was on the faculty at the University of Chicago.

Now with a growing family they wanted to live in a desirable community with good schools somewhere on the south side of Chicago. The Woodlawn region had degenerated, was decaying and had become unacceptable. Hyde Park was staid and with a somewhat elderly community although still desirable. The South Shore, however, was a relatively young, dynamic, growing community and that is where they chose to live, provided that an apartment could be located.

In April 1947, Bernie's sister, Tena, who was very active in the real estate business at that time and acquainted with the housing market, found out that an apartment of a friend of hers was going to be vacated in a three-story building in the South Shore area of Chicago, adjacent to the South border of Jackson Park. She was able to get the owners to rent the apartment to Bernie and Rhoda for which they were most appreciative. However, it took one-thousand dollars in cash[1] (under the table) to get access to that apartment. Although Bernie and Rhoda's resources were not great at that time, they wanted to have their own place to live, so the apartment seemed like a good investment. When Bernie, Rhoda and Gerry left the senior Sarnats, to make up a little for the loss of their leaving, they gave them a canary in a cage, to which Bernie's mother became quite attached.

Bernie's two siblings and several of Rhoda's family as well as other mutual friends lived in this area. The Illinois Central Railroad suburban service and bus transportation were excellent. On 71st Street between Jeffrey and South Shore Drive, was an excellent full service business and shopping center. For Bernie, the University of

Illinois Medical Center was about 12 miles away, his office down-town was about 8 miles away, and the hospitals were from three to six miles away from where he lived. Sometimes Bernie would do surgery at one of the hospitals, drive home, have lunch, leave the automobile for Rhoda and take the Illinois Central back downtown to his office.

However, winter was difficult. At home, only street parking was available and sometimes the best parking space was three blocks away. The snow, the ice, and freezing temperatures made driving a serious problem. One incident that Bernie recalled while commut-ing home on the Outer Drive was as follows: There was a slight incline at 31st Street. Because of the ice on the roadway, a car slipped back on the incline, hitting another car, which caused a chain reaction. Such incidents would delay Bernie's getting home from 30 minutes to more than an hour. In another incident, Bernie had an emergency call at about 2 am and went to Michael Reese Hospital, which was at 29th Street, and the Outer Drive. On the way, it had just begun to snow. After Bernie had finished his sur-gery around 5 am, he found that all traffic had stopped because of the extreme amount of snow. Transportation was at a standstill. This was in the early 1950's, and the women in labor were being transported by helicopter for delivery of their babies. Therefore, Bernie had to leave his automobile there. Fortunately, the Illinois Central Railroad suburban surface service was still functioning. So, Bernie walked over to the 31st Street Station to take the train back home. The next day he took the Illinois Central Railroad back to Michael Reese and retrieved his automobile.

Bernie and Rhoda were delighted to have their own three-story walk-up apartment and it was here where Joan was born in 1948. Slowly, over the course of a year or two they furnished the apart-ment. The day before Thanksgiving in 1947, they also hired as housekeeper, a wonderful mature nineteen year-old black woman by the name of Emma Gilmore who was attractive and very pleas-ant and intelligent; Rhoda wanted to go back to work and re-establish her professional career. Emma stayed with the family until the Sarnats relocated to California. She was a most unusual woman who did a wonderful job of taking care of the family and especially the children. They offered her a position in Los Angeles after they had been there for a year and were reasonably well established again. However, Emma was in great demand and had accepted employment with one of the friends of the Sarnats.

Gerry, at two years and nine months started nursery school and took to it very well. At that age he was already displaying precociousness as well as getting into things.

When Joan was three years old (1951) and already well adjusted in nursery school, Rhoda decided to go back to work half-time; that is when she joined the United Charities of Chicago. She became an Assistant District Supervisor as well as supervising master degree students from the University of Chicago, School of Social Service Administration.

So Bernie and Rhoda lived quite contently in this middle-class South Shore neighborhood. A number of their friends lived nearby. Bernie's brother and sister had apartments just a few blocks away. Rhoda's mother, Florence, had moved in with her sister Minnie. She lived several blocks away and would be over every Tuesday for dinner. After Bernie's mother died in 1951, his father moved to South Shore and would also frequently join them for Tuesday dinners. In June of 1951, Bernie's parents celebrated their fiftieth wedding anniversary with the family-at-large and friends — some 100 in attendance (Fig. 16).

Bernie's father had retired from his drugstore business in 1949 and he and Fanny went to their summer home in Paw Paw Lake, Michigan. In August 1951, Bernie's mother, now aged 71, had a coronary attack and was hospitalized. Bernie came up the next day to the small fifteen-bed hospital in Watervliet, Michigan. While better care may have been available in Chicago, a hundred miles away, the trip by ambulance was too risky, so within a day or two she died of an acute coronary. She was brought back to Chicago and buried in the Sarnat family plot. This was the first experience of a death in the immediate Sarnat family. They had celebrated their fiftieth wedding anniversary just a few months before.

Bernie and Rhoda had a modest social life during this decade in Chicago. They would see their numerous friends. As many of the couples played bridge this led to playing bridge every Friday night. As Bernie's work at the University of Illinois and his private practice kept him busy, he gave up bridge; and much to Rhoda's regret she did also. In spite of a very busy career, Bernie always tried to be home for dinner by six o'clock every night.

When Gerry was five years old, he was enrolled in the O'Keefe grammar school, which was just a block or so away. Interestingly, one day his kindergarten teacher aware that his name was Gerard Sarnat, focused on the Gerard name and asked if his mother, by any chance, happened to be Rhoda Gerard. It turned out that she had had Rhoda as a student some thirty years before at the same school! Gerry was quite bright and showed it early. Joan also displayed brightness as she followed not only in Gerry's footsteps but also displayed, fortunately, independence. Both youngsters were fun to watch as they were growing up. Both became engaged early in a variety of activities.

In the early 1950's television was something new in the home. A favorite Sunday afternoon program for both Gerry and Joan was the Super Circus show with Mary Hartline where she "led" the orchestra — her long blond tresses and short skirt in prominent display. At that time a cousin of Rhoda's, George Barnard, was dating Mary Hartline. He eventually married her and then divorced her. Knowing Mary, the Sarnat's invited her over for dinner. When she arrived, Gerry at that time about seven years old was so surprised and overwhelmed to see his TV "heroine" that he ran into his bedroom and stayed there throughout Mary's visit.

Bernie and Rhoda lived in this walk-up apartment until December 1955 when they decided to move to California.

Chapter 22

PRACTICE OF PLASTIC AND RECONSTRUCTIVE SURGERY IN CHICAGO (1946–1956)

Although Bernie had been offered a full-time position at the University of Illinois, Chicago, he also wanted to spend half his time in the private practice of plastic and reconstructive surgery. But after World War II finding office space was just as difficult as finding an apartment. For the decade that he was in Chicago, Bernie was able to finally move in with a dermatologist by the name of Paul Weichselbaum, a fine man, with whom Bernie shared office space at 104 South Michigan Boulevard.

The Weichselbaum's had four sons and the two families became very good friends. About 1958 or so, after Bernie had left Chicago for California, Paul died of a heart problem. One of his sons, Ralph, whom Bernie saw growing up, is now an internationally known radiation-oncologist and head of the department at the University of Chicago. At a later date, Bernie would consult personally with him when he was faced with a carcinoma of the prostate, but that will be taken up later.

Practicing Plastic Surgery in Chicago

Bernie would be in the office three afternoons a week and doing surgery two or three days a week. Bernie was on the staff at Michael Reese Hospital and also had staff privileges at two smaller hospitals,

Woodlawn and Chicago Memorial. The chiefs of staffs at both hospitals had been former residents or staff members at the Department of Surgery of the University of Chicago, and Bernie knew them both well and they readily welcomed him to their staffs.

When Bernie first returned to Chicago, he received privileges at University Hospital where he had been an assistant in general surgery under Marshall Davison. So Bernie received immediate privileges there and performed a moderate number of surgeries until Dr. Davison suddenly died of a heart attack in 1947, a tragic loss.

While still in St. Louis, Bernie and Rhoda would go to the records room at Barnes Hospital on Sunday mornings to transcribe the procedures used on the 25 patients that he had operated on earlier. These transcripts included a complete history and physical examination, as well as plastic and reconstructive surgical problems, surgical procedures utilized, postoperative course results and pre- and postoperative photographs. Specifically, these procedures involved surgery to repair various facial fractures and soft tissue injuries, removal of tumors, neck dissection, restoration of scalp flaps to cover a skull defect, face lifts, nasal plastic surgery, reconstruction of cleft lip and palate, eyelid plastic surgery, breast reductions and breast lifts, abdominoplasty, skin grafting to cover burns, etc.

These records from St. Louis were brought with him to Chicago and would then be used to document his plastic surgery skills. Subsequently, they were submitted to the American Board of Plastic Surgery as part of the requirements for certification. In addition, Board certification also required a written examination, an oral examination and a practicum. In July 1946, he took the full-day written examination on plastic surgery.

Later that year he had to operate on three patients, each of whom presented a different challenge, while being observed by Dr. Wallace Stephenson from Grand Rapids, Michigan and Dr. Gordon New from the Mayo Clinic in Minnesota, both members of the Board of Plastic Surgery. The surgeries involved about four hours of operating time. Afterwards, Bernie and Drs. New and Stephenson spent an afternoon at the office of Dr. Sumner Koch, who was Professor of Surgery at Northwestern University Medical School, an outstanding hand surgeon and also a member of the Board of Plastic Surgery. Because Bernie knew that Dr. Koch was going to be monitoring and conducting the oral exam in part, he studied extensively in the hope that he would be able to demonstrate that he was reasonably knowledgeable on hand surgery. He also knew that Dr. Wallace Stephenson was an ear, nose and throat plastic surgeon, while Gordon New was an oral and plastic surgeon and thought it likely that both probably knew little about hand surgery.

Sure enough, in the afternoon, Dr. Koch started conducting the examination. He presented a patient with a hand problem. He first turned to Gordon New and asked him what he knew about the patient being presented. Dr. New, of course, did not know anything about hand problems. Koch then turned to Wallace Stephenson and asked, "What can you tell us about this patient?" Stephenson did not know a thing. Koch then turned to Bernie and asked, "Sarnat, you tell me something about it". Bernie saw it was a difficult case and while he knew something about it, he felt quite uneasy as Koch had just embarrassed these two outstanding plastic surgeons in front of him. Nevertheless, Bernie answered as best as he could. By then, Bernie felt he was in trouble. The afternoon eventually ended and everyone dispersed. Bernie then waited for the results and after a month or so of worry, he was notified that he had passed the Boards. In 1947, he became a full-fledged Board-certified plastic surgeon.

Plastic surgery and reconstructive surgery deals with the repair reconstruction or replacement of physical defects of form or function involving the skin, musculoskeletal system, cranio-maxillofacial structures, hand and other extremities, breast and trunk, and external genitalia. It uses aesthetic surgical principles not only to improve undesirable qualities of normal structures but also in all reconstructive procedures as well. It is performed on abnormal structures of the body, caused by birth defects, developmental abnormalities, trauma, injury, burns, infection, tumors or diseases.

Special knowledge and skill in the design and surgery of grafts, flaps, free tissue transfer and replantation is necessary. Competence in the management of complex wounds, the use of implantable materials, and tumor surgery is also required. Plastic surgery has been prominent in the development of innovative techniques such as microvascular and cranio-maxillofacial surgery, liposuction and tissue transfer. The foundation of surgical anatomy, physiology, pathology and other basic sciences is fundamental to this specialty. Competency in plastic and reconstructive surgery implies a special combination of basic knowledge, surgical judgment, technical expertise, ethics and interpersonal skills to achieve satisfactory patient relationships and problem resolution.[1]

The first two individuals to become Board certified in plastic surgery by examination were Wayne Slaughter who practiced in Chicago and a surgeon, Herbert Conway, in New York at Cornell University. They were the very first to take the examinations in 1942. Previous to that, about 75 to 100 were grandfathered in as they represented "the establishment" at that time. In 1947, Bernie was one of six to be Board certified by examination as described above.

Some Noteworthy Surgery Cases

Bernie recalled that among the several outstanding patients that he had in his private practice while in Chicago, two in particular stood out. It was around April of 1955, he had been called into an out-lying hospital by a pediatrician who had been taking care of two burned children for about a month. Treatment involved dressing their wounds daily, hoping that they would heal by epithealiazation and scar formation. When Bernie walked into the room of these two children, a brother and a sister, they began crying vigorously at the sight of doctors. This was understandable as changing their dressing was a very painful procedure. The children had been burned when the son put a match to his father's gas tank to see whether there was any gasoline in there. Indeed, he found out that there was. His five-year-old sister, who was fond of her brother and followed him around, was looking over his shoulder. Checking these children, Bernie found that about 30% of the boy's body was burned and slightly more of the girl's body. They were emaciated, losing fluids through open infected areas and generally declining in health. While they were not close to death, they were not in very good condition.

Bernie immediately transferred them to Michael Reese Hospital and spent the next three days doing intensive pre-operative preparation for them, which meant getting the wounds clean and giving them fluids. He brought them back to health as best he could and then spent the entire day from seven in the morning until five that evening, grafting their skin. Bernie probably devoted four to five full days to save these children. This was done by taking skin from areas that had not been burned. While there was some scarring, it was amazing how well the wounds eventually healed. By December of 1955, these children were well-healed and could be transferred to another plastic surgeon as Bernie was heading for California.

At the time of surgery, the father and mother wanted to know how much it was going to cost. Bernie indicated that the issue was saving the children. They indicated they would be willing to take on another mortgage but Bernie said that would not be necessary. Whatever they could afford to pay would be fine. Therefore, over the following months, they did pay some moderate fees. Nevertheless, they were very grateful to Bernie first for saving their children's lives and rehabilitating them, and second for being so understanding with the financial matters. Since then Bernie regularly received Christmas cards from them and they would burn hundreds of candles, a Catholic custom, in honor of Bernie. They were very faithful for years after that. Around 1965, the older son visited Bernie in California at his Beverly Hills office and initially confided that he was planning to become a priest. However, on a later visit, he indicated that he was not going to be a priest after all. He came in with his lady friend and indicated that they were getting married. His sister had moved to Miami, Florida and held an important job there in a city department. She did quite well. They both had survived their burns to lead perfectly normal lives.

When the parents were celebrating their 25th wedding anniversary, the children asked them what they wanted as a gift. The parents said that they would like to have dinner with Dr. and Mrs. Sarnat in Beverly Hills. So they flew out and they all had dinner together. Bernie then learned that the father was Jewish and the mother was Catholic; the children were raised Catholic. The family kept up with Bernie but eventually the mother died. Bernie indicated that he had not been in touch with the father for the last five or so years.

An interesting side note is that the resident who assisted Bernie in 1955 later told him that he was not interested in surgery. He was interested in psychiatry. It turned out that some years later he became a very prominent psychoanalyst who now practices in Beverly Hills. Whenever he meets Bernie, he reminds him of the many hours they spent together skin grafting these children.

Another interesting patient was an unusual woman who while living in Manila, Philippines during World War II, became a captive of the Japanese. When the American armed forces attacked Manila later in the war, this patient was severely burned. The American doctors did some emergency skin grafting at the time. She came to Bernie, however, in about 1950 for more definitive treatment. Among her various interests was stamp collecting. She had collected all the postage stamps printed during the occupation and organized them into booklets. When she learned that Bernie's wife, Rhoda, was also a stamp collector, she presented her with one of these highly desirable, rare and unusual booklets.

Some years later when Bernie and Rhoda traveled to the Far East in 1966, they stopped off in Manila and spent a lovely day with this former patient where they were handsomely entertained. It was a great reunion.

In October 1955, Bernie was invited to an organizational meeting of a new research society in plastic and reconstructive surgery. Milton Edgerton who was chief of plastic surgery at Johns Hopkins medical school in Baltimore, was one of the organizers. He and Robin Anderson, a plastic surgeon at the Cleveland clinic, proposed the formation of an organization that is today known as the Plastic Surgery Research Council. The carefully selected founding members were all colleagues interested in basic research in plastic and reconstructive surgery. No one west of Texas was included. Bernie chaired the third meeting of the Plastic Surgery Research

Council held in Los Angeles. Today it is a distinguished and vital organization.

At that time Bernie was busily involved studying the transplantation of one of the relatively simpler tissues, cartilage. Joseph Murray of the Harvard Medical School, another founding member, was deeply involved in the transplantation of the kidney, a complex organ. Bernie, while talking with Murray, commented that he was starting with a less complex tissue and as he learned more he would proceed to more complex ones. He wished Murray well. Some 35 years later in 1990, Joseph Murray was awarded the Nobel Prize for his fundamental work on kidney transplantation.

After moving to Beverly Hills, California, Bernie returned to Chicago two or three times in 1956 to see several patients and complete certain surgical procedures. In addition he spent time at the University of Illinois winding down programs still in need of completion. The next chapter focuses on Bernie's academic career in Chicago.

Chapter **23**

PROFESSOR OF ORAL AND MAXILLOFACIAL SURGERY AND PLASTIC SURGERY (1946–1956)

Bernie had been reasonably certain that in coming back to Chicago, an opportunity would present itself at the University of Illinois in terms of academia and research. Now the focus is on the ten years at the University of Illinois, College of Dentistry, College of Medicine and Graduate School from 1946 to 1956 where he was invited to become head of the Department of Oral and Plastic Surgery. During these ten years, the Dental School had developed an international reputation. When Bernie was invited to become the full-time head of the Department, he compromised by saying no to full-time as he wanted to also be in the private practice of plastic and reconstructive surgery half time.

Dr. Moorehead who was Bernie's predecessor had died in the 1940's. He was a long-time faculty member and had been active at the initiation of the undergraduate program in the 1920's. This undergraduate program was in existence and fully operating since that time. Drs. Eli Olech and Henry Droba were running the outpatient clinic and also giving some of the lectures to the undergraduate dental students in their third and fourth years. Ms. Rieke, the nurse, was invaluable in helping run the Department.

When Bernie was still a student and took the Oral Surgery course in 1939, Dr. Frederick B. Moorehead was the head of the

Department. One of the courses in the undergraduate program at that time involved a series of operative clinics once a week in the large operative auditorium where he might be demonstrating the taking out of a third molar. At that time literally nothing could be seen, the students heard even less and seemingly learned nothing. To Bernie it was a total waste of time. No formal lectures were involved. In contrast, in the outpatient clinics with Drs. Olech and Droba, however, he did receive the fundamentals dealing with dental extraction and the treatment of the occasional fractured jaw.

Development of the Graduate Program

When Bernie came in as head of the department, his main purpose was to maintain that which was good and build upon it. At that time there were no graduate or postgraduate activities at all in the Department and, of course, there were no graduate students. This was an area, in which Bernie had some expertise and felt that such programs could be successfully developed. Thus, among the various activities that Bernie undertook at the University of Illinois, several eventually attracted national and international attention.

Bernie finally accepted in his three-year graduate program two outstanding first-year students who were going to do basic research related to oral and maxillofacial surgery as well as become active members in the Department. The first two students accepted were Dr. Gans and Dr. Laskin. Dr. Benjamin Gans, whom Bernie had had as a senior student when he was teaching at St. Louis University College of Dentistry, was outstanding. Dr. Daniel Laskin was also an outstanding student. Together, they began a series of active research programs. Dr. Gans' particular project was studying the growth at the five facial sutures in the monkey for which he was eventually awarded a masters degree. This work received recognition from the orthodontic world and was eventually published in the *American Journal of Orthodontics*. Dr. Gans went on to become a member of the Department of Oral and Maxillofacial surgery at Northwestern University and subsequently head of the Department at Michael Reese Hospital in Chicago and had quite an outstanding career.

Dr. Laskin proved to be a very unusual student who became interested in problems that were more difficult. As one of Bernie's early interests was in cartilage, he introduced Dr. Laskin to the study of the metabolism of cartilage and cartilage grafts. Dr. Laskin then worked with Dr. Bain at the Neuropsychiatric Institute who initially introduced him to the technique used for monitoring the metabolism of cartilage and cartilage grafts i.e., the use of the Warburg respirometer. Dr. Laskin eventually spent his third year as a resident at Cook County hospital in Oral Surgery. He then joined Bernie's staff. In subsequent years after Bernie had resigned from the University of Illinois and left for California, Dr. Laskin eventually became head of the Department taking over Bernie's position.

So in essence, this was the beginning of the graduate program and subsequently every year or two, Bernie accepted additional students until a year or two before leaving for California. Some of those other students of note were Dr. Robinson, Dr. Selman, Dr. Akamine, Dr. Rosen, and Dr. Roy, all of whom went on to publish papers in the *American Journal of Anatomy, Anatomical Record* or other refereed journals. Each obtained an M. S. degree. The graduate students took a series of courses such as mathematical biophysics, statistics, anatomy, etc. In addition to establishing the graduate program, he also became a member of the Plastic Surgery department in the Medical School.

Bernie also became quite active himself; publishing a number of important basic science publications in the emerging field of craniofacial and bone biology.[1-11]

Research Awards in Plastic Surgery

In addition, Bernie independently conducted research programs. Two in particular deserve mention. One was the experiment on effects of mandibular condylectomy on young monkeys. This proved to be a very innovative experiment, one that had never been done before and the bony changes that occurred were quite impressive.

While this work was in progress, he learned that for the first time a series of prizes were being awarded for research in plastic surgery by the American Society of Plastic and Reconstructive Surgeons. With this prize in mind, during the summer of 1949 while Bernie's family was staying at the summer home of his parents at Paw Paw Lake, Bernie would come back to the University of Illinois on Monday and work for two or three days preparing specimens, examining them to determine the findings, photographing them and beginning to write a manuscript. He submitted this material at an international competition. The first prize went to a Chinese National from mainland China, the second prize went to a United States citizen (Bernie), third prize went to an Argentinean and the fourth prize went to a citizen of the of UK. As a result, Bernie was invited to present his material at the annual meeting of the American Society of Plastic and Reconstructive Surgeons in Mexico City. The material was published in the *Journal of Plastic and Reconstructive Surgery* in 1950. This was known as the junior award for young scientists.

A second research experiment that Bernie worked on was the production of complete surgical clefts of the hard and soft palate in young monkeys. He studied the effects of this experiment and submitted a paper in 1957 for the senior research award in plastic surgery. He received this award in 1958 in San Francisco. This was the first time that someone had won both the junior and senior research awards in plastic surgery.

Bernie was also involved in three large educational programs, one on the temporomandibular joint, another one on cancer of the mouth and face, and a third one dealing with the international telephone courses, which are described in the next sections.

Temporomandibular Joint Problems

A major research area that involved Bernie, dealt with the temporomandibular joint. In the late 1940's, there were very few well-organized programs and the literature was woefully inadequate. Given Bernie's background, practitioners not knowing what to do in the care of these temporomandibular joint problems, would send their patients to Bernie at the University of Illinois. Bernie himself initially knew very little about this difficult clinical problem. As a result, he organized a postgraduate course. Dentists, orthodontists, oral surgeons, orthopedic surgeons, ear nose and throat doctors, plastic surgeons, and other specialists who had an interest in the temporomandibular joint attended these sessions. There were actually six 2-hour sessions of those lectures, each a month apart. Bernie brought in some outstanding basic scientists and clinicians to present the material. They included Drs. Harry Sicher, Peter Weinmann, Arnold Zimmermann and Allen Brodie. Bernie gave some of the lectures. The attendance at these very popular lectures was over 100 each time. At the last meeting, there was a demand for a more detailed organized publication.

As a result, the first edition of *The Temporomandibular Joint* was published in 1951.[12] This was followed by a second edition in 1964,[13] a third edition in 1980[14] and reprinted in Japanese in 1983,[15] and a fourth edition in 1991.[16] The concept of the book was to stress the basic science aspects and how they related to the clinical application of treatment of temporomandibular joint problems. Although a number of books exist today on the subject, none is comparable to this one. This was also the subject for one of the long-distance telephone courses. Subsequently, a clinic was organized for the diagnosis and treatment of these problems. At one time, the textbook was even cited in *Gray's Anatomy*.[17]

During this period a number of articles were also published.[18–23] Additional publications at that time were.[24–29]

Oral and Facial Cancer

Another major undertaking that involved Bernie was the organization and teaching of the subject of oral and facial cancer. While a resident at Cook County Hospital in Chicago (and later on the attending staff), Bernie saw a number of patients with oral and facial cancer. His experience was further enhanced during his three years in St. Louis where a number of patients were being treated for head and neck cancer. This extensive background indicated a need for a cancer program for dentists and Bernie was now well equipped to organize and teach the subject not only to dental but also to medical and postgraduate students and, of course, utilizing the telephone programs to be described subsequently. In addition to the lectures, a set of 35mm slides on oral and facial cancer was also made available. Eventually this slide set was also duplicated in conjunction with the Clay Adams Company,[23] so that the something like a hundred slides was made available to those who wanted them in addition to the eventual book that came out.

The outline for this book was born during a two-week vacation with the Schours and Sarnats going to Lake Columbine, Colorado in 1948. Dr. Schour and Bernie produced the first edition of *Oral and Facial Cancer* in 1950.[20] This book was reprinted in 1953[24] and eventually translated into Portuguese[28] and published in Brazil in 1956. It was used as a textbook in some of the dental schools. A second edition was published in 1957.[29]

Long Distance Telephone Courses

Bernie had already begun to give this course on oral and facial cancer to the senior dental students. This led to the original telephone courses. Back in about 1948 with the help of a dental alumnus, Saul Levy, who lived in Scranton, Pennsylvania. Bernie arranged to have a two-hour session course, one going to Scranton, Pennsylvania and the other to New Iberia, New Orleans, the reason being that Saul Levy knew someone there to serve as organizer. The two of them, Schour and Levy, arranged with the telephone company to send these sessions via telephone. What they did was to have a series of lecturers and sent their slides previously to the two cities — Scranton, Pennsylvania and New Iberia, Louisiana. So when the speaker called for a specific slide, it was shown at the University of Illinois as well as simultaneously at the other two places. This proved to be a learning experience and became quite successful once the kinks had been worked out. They found that after the first hour that they had not obtained New Iberia on the phone. The reason was that New Iberia was in a different time zone from the one that Bernie and his co-workers were in. They adjusted the difference when they got into the second hour. This was a one-time two-hour program on the subject of oral and facial cancer. In 1949, The Illinois division of the American Cancer Society was so impressed with the program that they asked Bernie to put on a series for five cities in the State of Illinois. As a consequence, he began the sessions in the five cities; this was the beginning of a much more expansive program. Dr. Levy now came in on this even more intensively. In fact, he moved to Chicago to help administrate this program. The enthusiastic response led to the engagement of full-time personnel and every year up to 1957, when television became popular, six such monthly two-hour programs, with a moderator, and five nationally recognized authorities were produced (Figs. 28 and 29).

These programs, aimed primarily at dental and medical subjects, were broadcast live. In advance, a 50 to 75-page glossy manual was sent out with each annual program. The contents included photographs of the speakers, outlines of their talk, brief summaries and selected illustrations. These manuals were so outstanding that they received national awards several times. This in turn received a tremendous response from the community, both locally and nationally, and even internationally, because at one time nearly every state in the union was receiving the program. This included Alaska as well as Hawaii. It was also going to the armed forces overseas.

American Telephone and Telegraph (AT&T) was in charge of the communications, which were sent to as many as 180 "classrooms" with a live attendance as high as 14,000 at one time. In addition, 35 mm slides, as many as 200 to 300, were also sent out in advance to be shown in each "classroom". These "classrooms" were meeting rooms in which 30–40 students would attend the ATT hookup, which provided sound and they would be able to see the accompanying projected slides. So the same slide would be shown simultaneously in each of the 180 "classroom" locations. Bernie served as a moderator for a number of the national — international telephone courses from 1949 to 1954.[18, 30-34] This was, for that time, a most unusual and highly successful experiment in long-distance telephone postgraduate education. The annual program was eventually terminated in 1956 with the increasing influence of television.

Ten years at the University of Illinois

During the ten years tenure while Bernie was at the University of Illinois, a number of new courses were developed at both the graduate and postgraduate level. These proved to be highly successful. At the graduate level he had gathered a number of devoted students several of whom became world renowned. Each week would be a departmental conference on Wednesday at noon. One week would be devoted to research in progress and research to be done and what critique could be given to the individual on the project so that they could sharpen their focus. A second week would be a seminar delivered by an outside speaker, a third week would be a business meeting, the fourth week, would be a review of literature and if there was a fifth week it would be an open session.

Of the many speaking engagements, that Bernie had during the 1946–1956 decade, a few stand out. He gave lectures at universities and organizations in the United States and abroad. One lecture in particular remains sharply in his mind. He was invited to give a series of talks on oral and facial cancer by the head of the State of Montana public health system. These were five evenings, each with a social hour followed by dinner and a one-hour lecture and discussion. Bernie was met at the Glendive Airport in eastern Montana on a beautiful warm, clear, and sunny Monday afternoon by the head of public health. This was in late November in 1948. That evening he spoke before a group of physicians and dentists. The next morning the head of the department of public health drove Bernie to Miles City and a second lecture was given. The same pattern was followed at Billings and Bozeman, Montana. The last lecture was given at Butte, Montana on Friday evening. During the social hour, someone mentioned that it had begun to snow.

After the talk, Bernie rushed to the airport because he had to be back in Chicago for surgery on Monday morning. When he arrived at the airport, it was already closed because of the large amount of snow. There was a bus leaving for Minneapolis at midnight and or possibly a train leaving the next morning at 10 am so he took the bus across Montana, North Dakota to Minneapolis. On the way, at any city with an airport, Bernie would telephone and check about any possible flights to Minneapolis or, hopefully, Chicago. There were no flights. He finally arrived to a cold, blustery, somewhat snowy Minneapolis about 6 pm on Saturday some 24 hours later. There was a possible flight to Chicago at 9 pm. Fortunately, Bernie was able to make this flight and arrived home at sometime after midnight tired, unshaven, disheveled but very happy to be home. He recovered on Sunday with his family and was in surgery Monday morning.

These were busy times and Bernie dealt with each of the programs. These included the graduate programs, the undergraduate and the postgraduate one. At the end of each academic year, they would have a departmental picnic. In addition, every year or two, Bernie would invite the professional staff to his home for dinner.

PEOPLE AND PLACES

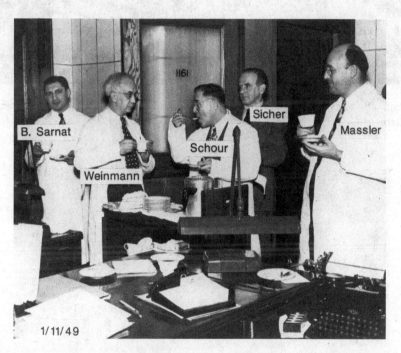

Fig. 27. 1949. Isaac Schour Birthday Party. 11th floor, 808 S. Wood Street, Chicago, Dental Histology Office and Laboratories.

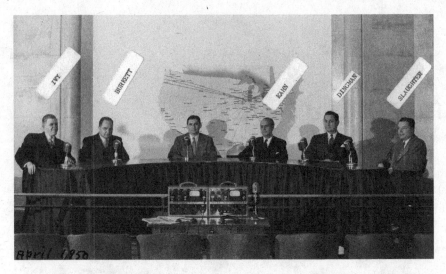

Fig. 28.   April 1950. University of Illinois Long Distance Telephone Course. Bernard G. Sarnat, Moderator.

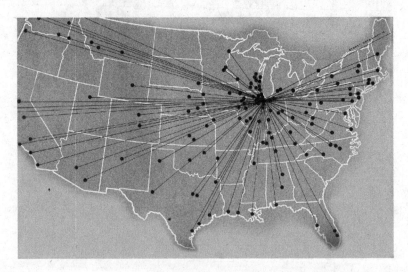

Fig. 29.   1951. University of Illinois Long Distance Telephone Course. Map showing some of the receiving groups in the United States.

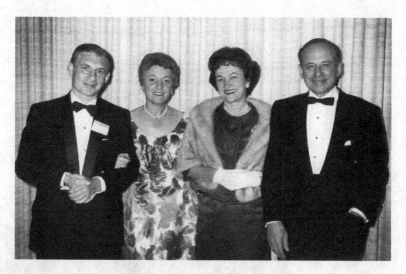

Fig. 30. 1957. Bernie and Rhoda and Mrs. Benjamin (Estelle) Graham and Benjamin Graham (Rhoda's first cousin). New Years Eve formal Dinner-Dance Party at 611 N. Maple Drive, Beverly Hills, California.

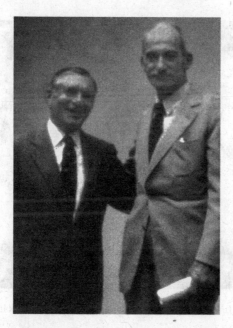

Fig. 31. 1964. Bernie and Paul Tessier (Father of Craniofacial Surgery) at UCLA, Los Angeles, California.

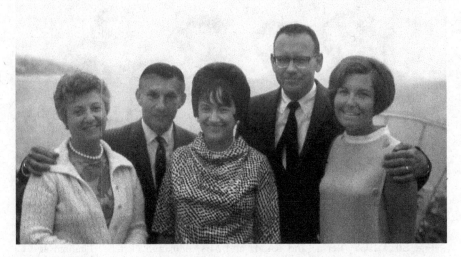

Fig. 32. 1966. Bernie and Rhoda and Mrs. Benjamin (Estey) Graham and Warren (former student of Benjamin Graham) and Susan Buffett. Emerald Bay, California.

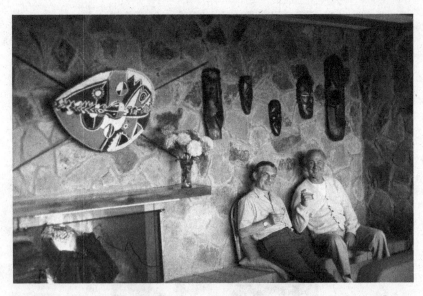

Fig. 33. 1969. Bernie and Irving Stone at William Holden's luxurious lodge in East Africa.

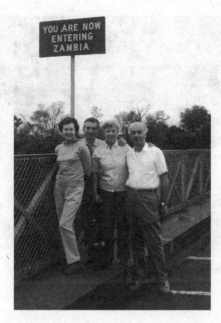

Fig. 34. 1969. The Sarnats and Irving Stones about to enter Zambia, East Africa.

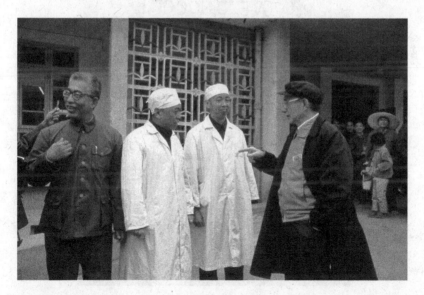

Fig. 35. 1979. Bernie after plastic surgery rounds outside hospital at Nanning, China.

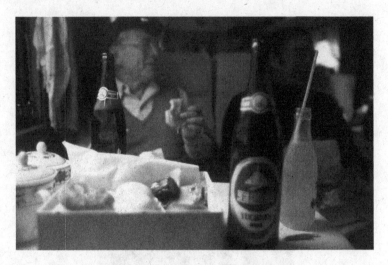

Fig. 36.   1979. Bernie enjoying lunch on train en route China.

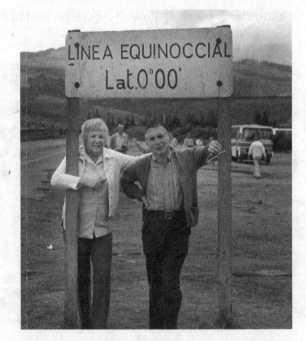

Fig. 37.   1980. Bernie and Rhoda in Ecuador at the equator.

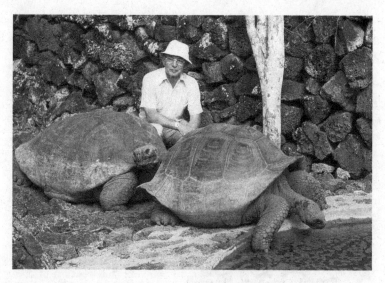

Fig. 38.   1980. Tortoises and Bernie on the Galapagos Islands.

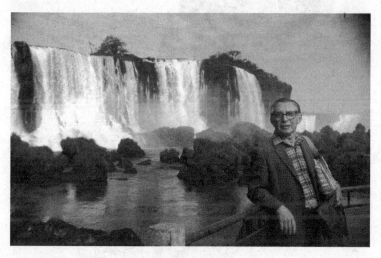

Fig. 39.   1981. Bernie at Iguaçu Falls, Brazil.

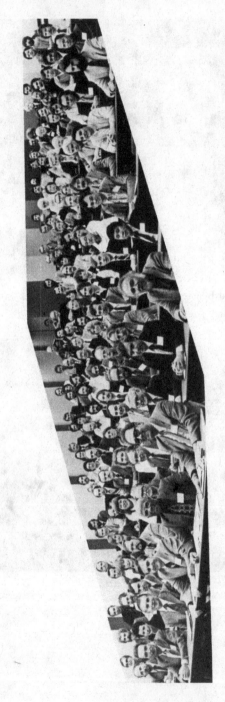

Fig. 40. 1982. International Bone Biology Conference at UCLA, Los Angeles, California. Bernie was a co-sponsor and is in the front row second from the left. The author is in the fourth row third from the left. More than 200 attended from 15 different countries and 15 different disciplines.

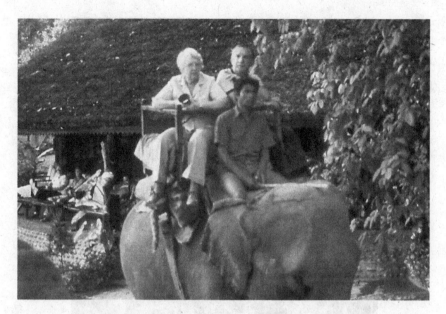

Fig. 41. 1985. Bernie and Rhoda riding an elephant in Nepal out hunting rhinocerouses with camera.
Note: Quality unfortunately degraded in the orginal.

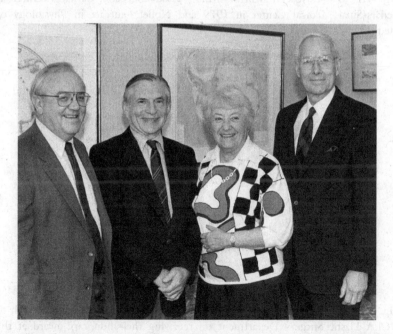

Fig. 42. 1988. Bob Roberts, Dean of University of Southern California, School of Social Work, Bernie and Rhoda and President Zumberge.

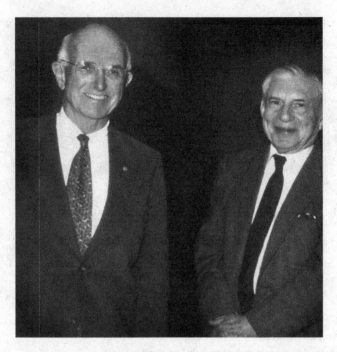

Fig. 43. 1994. Joseph Murray, M.D., Plastic Surgeon. Sarnat Lecturer at Cedars-Sinai Medical Center in 1979 and Nobel Laureate in Physiology or Medicine in 1990 and Bernie.

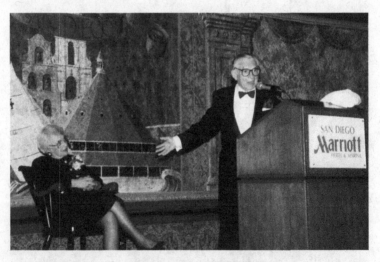

Fig. 44. 1994. Bernie introducing Rhoda before giving acceptance speech to UCLA Plastic Surgery Department on receiving their honorary award at the American Society of Plastic and Reconstructive Surgery Annual Meeting in San Diego, California.

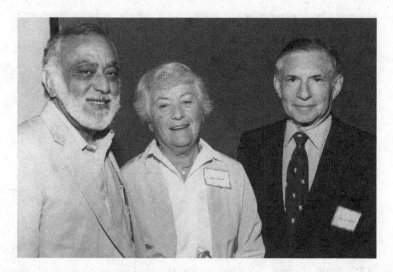

Fig. 45. 1994. Moshe Manny President of Tel Aviv University and Rhoda and Bernie.

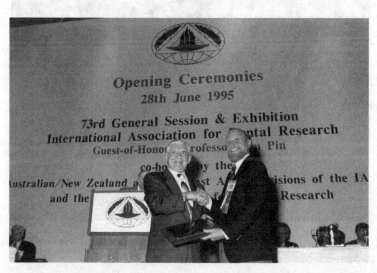

Fig. 46. 1995. Bernie receiving the International Craniofacial Biology Award in Singapore at the International Association for Dental Research Meeting.

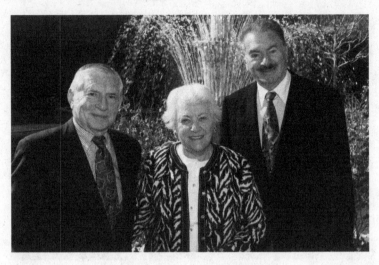

Fig. 47. 1996. Bernie and Rhoda with Manny Finemann (personal friend), National President of the City of Hope, Duarte California.

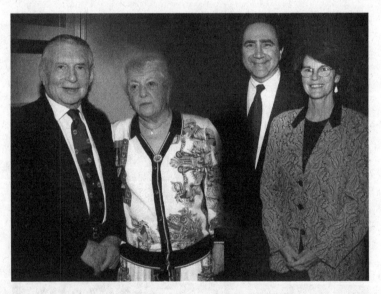

Fig. 48. 1998. The Sarnats with the President of the University of Chicago, Hugo Sonnenschein and his wife.

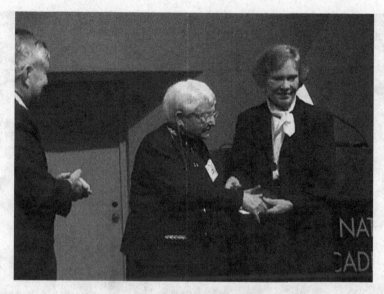

Fig. 49. 2000. The Sarnats with Rosalynn Carter. Institute of Medicine, Washington, D.C.

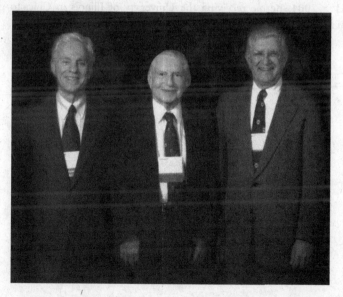

Fig. 50. 2003. Bernie in Chicago, receiving the University of Chicago at large Achievement Award. On the left, Atkinson, President of the University of California on the right, Randel, President of the University of Chicago.

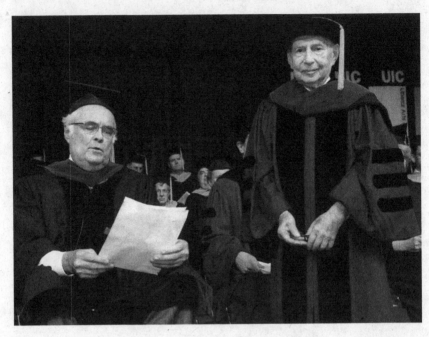

Fig. 51.   2004. Bernie receiving the University of Illinois in Chicago general Alumni Achievement Award in Chicago.

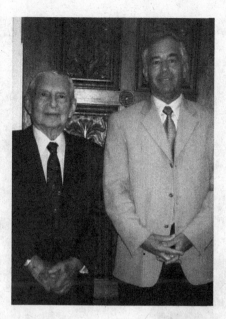

Fig. 52. 2006. Bernie with Jehuda Reinharz, President of Brandeis University.

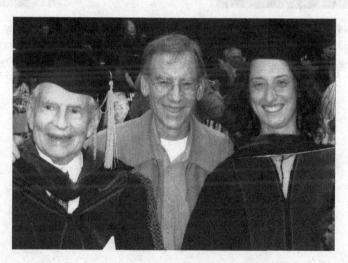

Fig. 53. 2007. Three generations of M.D.'s. From the right: Zoe Sarnat Aron, UCLA School of Medicine, 2007; Gerard D. Sarpat, Stanford University School of Medicine, 1972; Bernard G. Sarnat, University of Chicago School of Medicine, 1937.

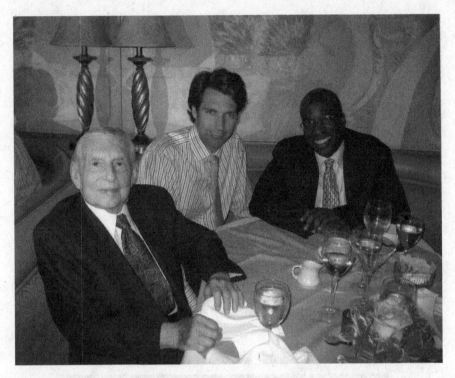

Fig. 54.   2007. Two holders of the Sarnat Chair in Craniofacial Biology. From the right: Russell Reid M.D., Ph.D., Division of Plastic Surgery, University of Chicago Pritzker School of Medicine; James Bradley, M.D., UCLA Division of Plastic Surgery, David Geffen School of Medicine; Bernard G. Sarnat, M.D.

Chapter 24

THE MOVE TO CALIFORNIA (1955)

Before discussing the move to California, a few introductory remarks are in order. Having spent a year (1936/1937) as an intern in Los Angeles, Bernie found that the allergies that bedeviled him in the Midwest were not present in Los Angeles. He had a great allergy-free year in Southern California. Because he also fell in love with the weather and the community, he stayed on after his internship for about a month or two to take the medical state board exam. Of course, from 1931 to 1936, Rhoda (then unknown to Bernie) had been living in Beverly Hills, which is a separate city surrounded by Los Angeles.

Now skipping on to 1946, when Bernie and Rhoda were ready to leave St. Louis, he inquired about the possibility of moving to Los Angeles to practice plastic and reconstructive surgery and, of course, to live there. Because of the initially negative responses to inquiries about moving to Los Angeles, the Sarnats had moved back to Chicago.

A primary reason for the eventual move to California was Bernie's and Gerry's seasonal allergies and asthma, which began in May with the blooming of the trees, grasses and weeds, and lasted until late September. The ragweed and asthma were particularly bad in August and September and became worse each year forcing the family to leave the Chicago area and go far to the north. This was but a continuation of the problem prior to 1946. Thus, the

Sarnats, in August and September, would leave the Midwest to avoid the problems.

When Joan was fifteen months old, in 1949, Rhoda and Bernie took her with them to the Upper Peninsula of Michigan along the southern border of Lake Superior and spent August and September there. They left Gerry, their son, with Bernie's parents at their summer home at Paw Paw Lake in western Michigan. Upon their return they found that to their utter dismay that Gerry was suffering from the same allergies as his dad, if not worse. For two or three years, the family would continue to go up to the Upper Peninsula to avoid in particular ragweed pollination. Finally, in 1953, it became increasingly clear that they could not stay much longer in the Midwest. Therefore, they had decided it was time to leave for a less allergic environment.

There were several other factors, less troubling, but they played roles as well. Bernie did a great deal of traveling within Chicago with living on the Southside and the University of Illinois being about twenty miles away on the Westside, while his private practice office was in the downtown area about eight miles away. In addition, the several hospitals that he used were scattered from three to fourteen miles away on the Westside and the Southside. Although all that driving was a problem in good weather, it was greatly exacerbated in the wintertime with freezing temperatures, the snow and ice, etc.

All the Sarnats were growing a bit weary of constantly fighting the winter elements. In addition, Bernie found that his work at the University of Illinois required more and more administrative time. He had less time for research and was devoting less time to his private practice. All in all, the Sarnats were ready to move, but where — to another Chicago area or perhaps elsewhere?

In the 1950's, what had been the ideal community of South Shore was beginning to show signs of deterioration. This had also occurred in the Woodlawn District in the 1920's and in Kenwood and Hyde Park areas in the 1930's. The decline was made apparent by the fact that the wonderful business street, 71st St., showed

signs of store vacancies with merchants leaving the area and apartments becoming increasingly available.

Rhoda and Bernie discussed at great length what to do. This
was a period when there was a flight to the suburbs, where housing was much preferred and the schools were generally excellent.
Many of their friends were moving to the North Shore of Chicago
and some to the very far Southside of Chicago. However, this was
impractical for Bernie since he had his connections at the
University of Illinois and his hospital affiliations were in Chicago as
well as his office so that all of those possibilities were ruled out.
Another consideration was the Westside suburb of Oak Park, which
was very close to Chicago. This was a long-term well-established
community but was not particularly appealing to either Rhoda or
Bernie. A fourth possibility was that of moving to one of the high-
rise buildings in Hyde Park along the Lake Shore. This neighborhood was not conducive particularly for the raising of children and
also did not appeal to either Rhoda or Bernie.

In view of the above problems, the thought arose of considering moving out of the Chicago area. With this idea in mind, they
began exploring the possibility of living in Miami, Florida, which
was ragweed pollen free. After spending August and September
1953 there, their feelings became negative toward this move. The
reason was that living there was not that pleasant. While the temperature did not rise above the high eighties, the humidity was so
high that it caused excessive perspiration and discomfort. They
would have to stay in the swimming pool or air conditioned room
to be comfortable. Additionally, there were swarms of insects. So
they decided that Florida was not a good choice after all. The
Sarnats then considered all the communities between San Diego,
California and Seattle, Washington and concluded that Los Angeles
was the most desirable place to live. It was also a place with which
both of them were familiar.

So in August of 1954, ostensibly on vacation, the four Sarnats
drove from Chicago to Los Angeles where they lived for a month.
On the way the family spent time at the Grand Canyon, Bryce and
Zion National Parks. It was hot driving (no air-conditioning in the

automobile) but the kids were promised a swimming pool at Zion. They could not wait to jump in the water, which was icy cold being fed by a mountain stream. Nevertheless, they enjoyed it. Then it was on to Las Vegas and Los Angeles.

Once in Los Angeles, the Sarnats renewed acquaintances and explored the possibility of living there with Bernie practicing and doing research. Bernie gave some lectures, checked out a variety of items, like office space, housing, hospital affiliations and the receptivity of another plastic surgeon in town. The responses from everyone concerned were very favorable. In addition, once they were in Los Angeles, Gerry and Bernie had no more problems allergy-wise. The family then flew back to Chicago with plans very likely to move to Los Angeles the following year but not before having a family discussion, which turned out positive with everyone in favor of the move.

Upon the return to Chicago, they began to make the necessary decisions regarding moving permanently to Los Angeles. These included terminating the lease of the apartment, disposing of unnecessary household items not required for the move, terminating the office lease, notifying patients, terminating Bernie's hospital appointments and his relationship with the University of Illinois.

While quite certain that the move to Los Angeles would take place, the Sarnats decided, nevertheless, to travel once more to Southern California to see if their decision was indeed the correct one. Because they now felt confident of their move, they purchased a second automobile, a new 1955, stick shift Chevrolet prior to the second trip in August and September of 1955. They then left this new (second) automobile in Los Angeles. Since Bernie had a meeting to attend in Los Angeles in October of 1955, having the car left there proved useful. They also started to look around for places to live.

Bernie flew back to Chicago with Joan a bit earlier and Rhoda returned with Gerry a bit later. In September 1955 Bernie tended his resignation at the University of Illinois and began procedures to stop seeing new patients and doing surgery in private practice.

With his resignation from the university, he gave up a full professorship, being head of the department, a pension and his appointments in the dental, medical and graduate schools as well as tenure. Although Bernie could have qualified for a pension if he had stayed on an additional nine months, the family was eager to move. Another important decision was to notify their housekeeper, Emma Gilmore, who had been with them since Thanksgiving of 1947. She was a wonderful, understanding, intelligent young black woman who helped raise their two children and took care of many of the family needs. They offered to hire her in California after a year and had made their adjustments, but she deferred and being in great demand by others, she accepted another position in Chicago.

On to Los Angeles

In early December of 1955, after having disposed of much of the belongings that were not wanted they arranged for shipment to Los Angeles of the rest of the household. Emma worked for the Sarnat's until the last evening in early December when they left for California. Emma helped Bernie and the movers get all the household furnishings into the van prior to the move. Emma will re-appear again later but that story will be deferred to a future chapter.

The four Sarnats then stayed overnight with Bernie's brother's family and the next morning, on a cold, crisp, and clear Sunday, in December 1955, for the third time in sixteen months, they drove again to Los Angeles, leaving Chicago with many fond memories and started on a new chapter of their lives. All four of them were quite enthusiastic about the new venture on the West Coast. So it was good-by Chicago and hello Los Angeles.

They traveled practically non-stop, being very eager to get to California and start life anew. In 1954 they had found a great motel, the Ashley Arms on Wilshire Boulevard in West Los Angeles. It had two bedrooms, a kitchenette, swimming pool and continental breakfast. They had stayed there earlier in August and also the previous year, so it was an ideal place. Fortunately, they were able to make reservations at the Ashley Arms again.

Bernie's program was planned to be similar to the one in February of 1946 when they arrived in Chicago. Once again the program was three-pronged. First, to establish the family in a desirable community, obtaining a home in a place where the schools were excellent. Next, was establishing a practice in plastic and reconstructive surgery. This meant locating an office, hospital connections and becoming known in the community at large. The final issue was becoming reestablished in regard to research, teaching and academia.

Soon after the Sarnats had settled down at the Ashley Arms and reconnected with their acquaintances, Rhoda and Bernie began looking for more permanent housing. The furniture was to arrive from Chicago in about three weeks and they thought that it would be nice if they had a somewhat permanent place to live to house the furniture. Consultation with friends, newspapers and realtors led to several leads, a couple of which were of interest. The Park La Brea housing complex (now known as Park La Brea Towers) was quite modern, desirable and centrally located. Bernie and Rhoda checked it out and found that two adjoining one-bedroom apartments were available. Their offer, however, was refused since they would not permit a 10-year-old boy and a seven-year-old girl to share the same bedroom. The next viable offer was in Brentwood. This was a delightful one-story apartment which was also highly desirable although the rent was a bit more than they were prepared to pay. This offer was also refused because children were not accepted.

Subsequently, while driving alone down Olympic Boulevard in Beverly Hills, Bernie noticed a "for rent" sign for an apartment. It was owned by a very nice elderly widow. The apartment was one of a three-apartment complex, which had a living room, dining room and kitchen downstairs, and two bedrooms upstairs. There were many additional positives. There was a two-car garage which took care of the two automobiles, she welcomed children and the rental was modest. Another big plus was that across the alley was the Beverly Hills-Beverly Vista grammar school. Bernie immediately brought Rhoda to see the apartment and as she fully approved of the choice, a one-year lease was signed. This was an ideal location. Thus, in spite of a busy period with all the arrangements that needed to be made, the children missed very little time from school especially since Christmas vacation also took place in December. The furniture arrived one week later. And thus they began to settle down in their new home in Beverly Hills.

The Sarnats knew that Rhoda's mother would be following them to Los Angeles from Chicago. They had asked her not to come until they were reasonably settled down. But, lo and behold, she announced that she would be arriving on December 30, 1955. So now during this very busy transition period, they also had to locate a place for her to live. Fortunately, they were able to find a very nice apartment-hotel, the Langham, at seventh and Normandy in Los Angeles. While a hotel, the apartment-like setting had a kitchenette, a beauty parlor and a small market within the complex. The residents were elderly and many were widows.

So the Sarnats began to settle down in their apartment on Olympic Boulevard, Beverly Hills. It was a wonderful year there and it gave both Rhoda and Bernie a chance to orient themselves to the city and its environs and allowing the children to adjust themselves to school.

One day, when Bernie came home to their new apartment on Olympic Boulevard, he found that Rhoda had acquired two cute little kittens. Rhoda had always wanted pets. Back in Chicago, she had had a dog, a small collie (sheltie), which proved to be quite neurotic and had to be returned to the owners. With the assistance of the kids, the kittens were named Tiger (because it had stripes) and Panther (because it was black). Panther loved to jump on and slide down the drapes, thereby tearing them. One day when Bernie came home, Panther jumped on Bernie's shirt, dug in his claws and tore it. That was the end of Panther. He was appropriately placed elsewhere with neighbors. Tiger, however, was more docile and lovable. He continued to live with the Sarnats until he died around 1967.

House Hunting

During the first six months in 1956, Bernie made two trips to Chicago for two reasons: (1) to have a follow up on patients that he operated on; and (2) to finish work at the University of Illinois. On one of those trips, Bernie noticed bright red blood during a bowel movement. He immediately called a close friend who had been his internist who examined Bernie. He did a proctoscopy. He showed Bernie bright red blood spots on his rectal glove hand and indicated to Bernie that a small hemorrhoid was probably the source of bleeding. However, this did not satisfy Bernie and he went to a very good friend of his who was a radiologist and had a barium enema. The report indicated that he had a normal colon. Bernie took the X-ray films back with him to California. This incident would lead to serious health consequences later on (taken up in Chapter 27).

With the children settled into their schooling, Bernie and Rhoda began house hunting. Each week, Rhoda would see several homes in Beverly Hills and then on the weekend, Rhoda would take Bernie to look at the three most desirable ones. Bernie would invariably find flaws in the homes that Rhoda had selected. This went on for many weeks and finally Rhoda in disgust said: "I don't think you really want to buy a home, so I am going to stop looking." After a while Bernie started looking himself and became much more knowledgeable about the housing market in 1956 in Beverly Hills. He wanted a home within walking distance from the school, a quiet neighborhood, a one-story home etc. A realtor showed him one home in the 500 block of North Canon Drive, a dilapidated, deserted home with World War I newspapers on the wall. Bernie commented that the home was not livable and the realtor responded by saying: "Doctor you're buying the land not the house." So for a few months the house hunting activities were rather diminished. Then in early September of 1956, out of the blue, Bernie received a telephone call from one of his cousins. He indicated that a widow was putting her home on the market in Beverly Hills and that they might want to take a look at it. Bernie went to see the home and to his surprise found that it was at 616 North Maple Drive in Beverly Hills, a prime area, and located directly across the street from the home of Benjamin and Estelle Graham, cousins of Rhoda's.

There were, of course, positives and negatives to buying this house. The positives won. It was a gracious Mediterranean style split-level with more than 3,000 square feet, with four bedrooms and four bathrooms and a very large living room with a cathedral ceiling. The kitchen, bathrooms and other areas were in need of extensive remodeling. Nevertheless, the place was immediately livable.

Chapter 25

PERSONAL LIFE IN BEVERLY HILLS

After moving into 616 North Maple Drive, Bernie and Rhoda hired a full-time housekeeper. With the children well placed in school, Rhoda began working as a psychiatric social worker at the Los Angeles Psychological Service Center (LAPSC) in 1958. At that time Rhoda accepted a severely psychotic patient for treatment. This patient was described in detail in Chapter 19.

The Sarnats also began an active social life, renewing old friendships and making new ones, in particular with the parents of two school friends of their children. They would hold small dinner parties for about 12 and, in addition, several large cocktail parties for upwards of 100 people. In 1957, Bernie hosted the Third Annual Plastic Surgery Research Council meeting in Los Angeles and invited the membership and guests to a cocktail party and sit-down dinner for some 65 people in their home (mentioned in more detail in Chapter 26).

North Maple Drive, Beverly Hills

Although Bernie and Rhoda knew that this was a desirable neighborhood to live in, there was much that they did not know of the area between Santa Monica and Sunset Boulevards. This was known as the "flats" because it was level. There were sidewalks and it was a great area for walking. The region north of Sunset Boulevard was hilly.

North Maple Drive was a three-block area between Santa Monica and Sunset Boulevard, containing the 500, 600 and 700 blocks.

The further north toward Sunset Boulevard one went, the larger and more expensive were the lots and the homes. Maple Drive was essentially a residential street that did not extend either north or south past Santa Monica or Sunset Boulevards. The beautiful trees bore leaves all year around. However, they were not maples but camphor trees. At one time Maple Drive had been written up in Holiday magazine as one of the prettiest streets in America. The Sarnat home on North Maple Drive was midway between Santa Monica and Sunset Boulevards.

Bernie and Rhoda soon learned of some of their prominent neighbors. Next door to the north lived Leo Robin, the songwriter. Just across the street lived Luella Parsons, the Hollywood columnist. Toward the south in the 600 block lived Barbara Rush, the actress. In the 700 block lived Diahann Carroll, the singer, Burns and Allen and the Ritz Brothers comedy teams and Irving Stone, the author, with his wife Jean.

Gerard and Joan Sarnat

Rhoda and Bernie were strong believers in public education and this was a primary reason for moving into Beverly Hills. When they enrolled the children in Beverly Vista grammar school in south Beverly Hills in January of 1956, the transition from Chicago's O'Keefe grammar school was not difficult. Beverly Vista School was attended by students from mostly middle-class homes. However, the transition from Beverly Vista to Hawthorne grammar school in north Beverly Hills, which was within walking distance from their new home, about three blocks away, was rather significant because most of the students now came from upper-middle-class homes. Bernie and Rhoda were a bit concerned about the values of some of the children attending Hawthorne but felt that their own children had been imbued enough with their parents' values that it was safe to transfer them to Hawthorne. Fortunately, they made friends with similar values. Both excelled academically and were at the top of their classes. In the eighth grade both children took advanced placement courses at Beverly Hills high school while still at Hawthorne Elementary, which was an eight year curriculum (there was no junior high or middle school then).

Both of the children were also involved in a number of activities. Gerry was active in Little League and served both as a first baseman even though he was left-handed, and as a pitcher. On one of the opposing teams was Jim Palmer, a player who was practically a one-man team. When he was pitching, every batter was struck out by him and no one got a hit. As a batter he would invariably hit a homerun. He eventually became an outstanding pitcher for the Baltimore Orioles and won the Cy Young award several times and was inducted into baseball's Hall of Fame. Joan's interests at that time included ballet, which she took quite seriously. She was also invited to appear on a children's television program (Fig. 17).

Both children attended Beverly Hills High School which at that time was rated among the top three high schools in the country academically. Gerry attended the high school from 1959 to 1963 and was again a top student. While president of the senior class, he would meet with the presidents of the other school classes and happened to meet a young woman who was president of the sophomore class (Lela Ziff) who eventually became his wife. Gerry graduated from Harvard College in 1967 majoring in English. He then attended Stanford medical school from 1967 to 1972. He married Lela, born in 1947, in 1969. She had obtained her Ph.D. in Child Development also from Stanford. Gerry then served a residency at Beth-Israel Hospital in Boston and also at Stanford. He is currently an internist with a social conscience. He has a happy marriage with a lovely wife and three children. The family was raised in Portola Valley, California. The oldest, a daughter, Zoe, born December 3, 1973, also attended Harvard and graduated as a theater art major. She met her future husband Elijah Aron while at Harvard and they were married in 2003. She has completed medical school at UCLA, is now a resident in psychiatry, and become a mother of Simon in 2006. The second, a son, Eli, born May 7, 1978, is earning his Ph.D. in entomology at UC Davis. The third daughter, Emme, born December 11, 1984, has graduated from UC Santa Barbara in 2007.

Joan also graduated from Beverly Hills High School in 1966. She was active in ballet and won the outstanding student award in dancing. She also participated in acapella and debate. In 1960 she appeared as a Page in the British Royal Ballet in the performance of Sleeping Beauty with Margo Fontaine in the lead when it toured Los Angeles. She graduated from Radcliffe-Harvard as a psychology major in 1970 and then attended the University of Michigan where she received her Ph.D. in clinical psychology in 1975. She met and married her husband David Hoffman in 1975 at the University of Michigan, where David was teaching. They were married in the Meadow at the University of Michigan by a psychological minister.

David received his bachelor's degree from the University of Rochester in 1966 and received his Ph.D. from Stanford in mathematics in 1972. They then moved to Amherst, Massachusetts where he eventually became a professor of mathematics at the University of Massachusetts. He obtained a considerable reputation in mathematics with his work on minimal surfaces. Joan had a private practice in psychotherapy and has since become a psychoanalyst known for her expertise in the relational approach to the supervision of therapy. They had two children while at Amherst. The older son, Jascha, born July 4, 1979, graduated from Harvard as a religion major in 2002 and is currently an editorial assistant at the New York Review of Books as well as a freelance writer in New York. His younger brother, Michael, born June 10, 1984, graduated from Harvard in 2006 as a philosophy major and is now in the Ph.D program in philosophy at the University of Pittsburgh. In the 1990's the family moved permanently to Berkeley, California.

The Benjamin Graham Era

The Sarnats finally settled into their home on North Maple Drive in Beverly Hills in December 1956. Although it had a number of shortcomings, it did have a number of pluses and one of those, of course, was living across the street from the Grahams. The relationship of the Grahams to the Sarnats is explained below (Fig. 30).

There were at least three world-famous members of Rhoda's family. The first was her half-brother Ralph Waldo Gerard, a neurophysiologist who had been nominated for the Nobel Prize on two occasions. The second was a first cousin by the name of Rita Auerbach who was probably the first woman elected to the British House of Commons. The third and probably the most famous of all was Benjamin Graham who was a first cousin of Rhoda's. He was the son of Rhoda's father's sister Dorothy Graham. He was known as the father of security analysis and as the Dean of Wall Street. He was also known as a successful investor in a variety of enterprises. He had published a number of papers and at least two important books: one was *The Intelligent Investor*, which was for the layperson and the other was *Security Analysis*, which was for the professional and became the bible for many investors.

Benjamin Graham's family had been well off until his father died. His mother, Dorothy, known to Rhoda as Aunt Dora, eventually lost their fortune because of bad investments and her lack of experience in running the fine China business established by her husband. So in about 1908, she and Ben and his two older brothers, Leon and Victor, were forced to move in with Rhoda's father's family, Maurice Gerard and his first wife, and their three children Helen, Ralph and Elsie. This was quite a household. Maurice and Ben developed a close intellectual relationship. Both of them were geniuses. Details about Benjamin Graham can be found in the book *Benjamin Graham: The Memoirs of the Dean of Wall Street* by Seymour Chatman (1996). There are also several other books about him and in which both Rhoda and Bernie are mentioned, including *Benjamin Graham on Value Investing* by Janet Lowe (1994).

Bernie first learned about Benjamin Graham in 1944 and met him in 1950, when Rhoda and Bernie gave a 75th birthday party for her mother Florence, and Ben came in from New York to Chicago to attend this affair. In 1951 Bernie was invited to make a presentation at the New York Academy of Medicine. This gave Bernie and Rhoda an opportunity to visit Ben Graham in his office. Ben invited them to his home in Scarsdale for Sunday dinner where

Bernie and Rhoda met Estelle Messing Graham (1913–1981), Ben's third wife, and their six-year-old son, Benjamin Graham Jr., for the first time. Their son seemed rather precocious.

When Rhoda's mother, Florence, came to Los Angeles in December 1955, she knew that Ben had just retired and was now living in Beverly Hills. Having known Ben and his first wife very well for many years in New York, she felt free to call upon him and renew their acquaintance.

In 1956, Ben Graham had decided to retire and he and his family had moved to 611 North Maple Drive, Beverly Hills, California. The Sarnats, quite independently and on their own, decided to leave Chicago and move to Los Angeles. By sheer coincidence Bernie and Rhoda purchased a home at 616 North Maple Drive, directly across the street from the Grahams! Estey, Rhoda (and Bernie) very soon became close, inseparable, personal friends. Every afternoon Estey and Rhoda would take a walk and have tea at 611. Estey was a warm, giving, generous and non-judgmental person. Bernie would sometimes join them after office hours. Their sons Benjamin, Jr. and Gerry became close friends and remain so to this day. Even their housekeepers, Lucy and Emma, became close friends. Warren and Susan Buffett would often come to consult with Ben (his mentor). So it was in 1958 that Bernie and Rhoda met the Buffetts for the first time. In 1959 the Sarnats invested, with Estey's encouragement, with Warren in his partnership MO-BUFF, the precursor to Berkshire Hathaway. A warm personal relationship ensued that has lasted throughout the years, even with the unfortunate death of Susan Buffet a few years ago (Fig. 32).

The Grahams, who entertained frequently, invited Rhoda and Bernie to their dinner parties, as well as to the Hollywood Bowl and the Dorothy Chandler Pavilion where they had superb boxes. Through the years, at various times, the Sarnats met a number of their guests at dinners at their home including: Vern Knudsen who was then chancellor at UCLA; Neil Jacoby and Harold Williams, subsequent Deans at Anderson Business School, UCLA; Irving Stone, author, and his wife Jean; Will and Ariel Durant, historians;

Byron Janis, world-famous pianist; Warren Buffett, a former student of Graham's; Charles Munger, a close friend of Warren Buffett; William Ruane, founder of the Sequoia Mutual Fund; Jack Skirball, investor and philanthropist, a high school friend of Graham, and his wife Audrey (whose father played a pivotal role at General Dynamics); Wilfrid Bion, a psychoanalyst from London; and Jules Stein's sister, Ruth Stein Cogan, who managed the MCA bond portfolio. After dinner, when the social chitchat began, Ben would disappear. He was not one for small talk and would retire to his study to work.

Warren Buffett not only had been a student of Ben's at Columbia University Business School, but had also worked for Ben in his New York office. He would periodically come out to Beverly Hills to consult with Ben about financial matters, the details of which were, of course, confidential. His wife, Susan, would always come along. She was charming, delightful and very personable. After Warren Buffett's meeting with Graham, they would come across the street to 616 North Maple Drive for a ping-pong tournament. Warren Buffett would usually be number one in the ping-pong round robin. Ben Graham was number two, Buz Graham would be number three, Gerry Sarnat number four, Rhoda number five, Bernie about number nine and Joan brought up the rear at number twelve. Estelle and Susie would not participate. Later, they would all have dinner at the Grahams.

Ben Graham played a role in a few other areas as well. Buz and Gerry belonged to the Beverly Hills Boy Scout Troop of which Glenn Ford, the actor, was scoutmaster. He had a father-son steak fry at his home and Buz accidentally dropped his steak into the fire. Ben Graham, who always had a practical solution available, immediately suggested that they all go to a steakhouse restaurant in Beverly Hills. He also had a practical solution to fulfill a requirement which the Scouts had to learn. This was the Morse code. He devised a system using the words "Coca-Cola" as mnemonic to assist them in learning the Morse code in short order. Bernie also became very close friends with another one of the fathers of the Scout troop. He was Manny Fineman, who eventually became national president of the City of Hope. Their friendship lasted for 50 years until his death in 2004 (Fig. 43).

Another of Ben's contributions was his Sunday morning classes for those children who did not belong to a church or temple. These were general discussions about the history of religions which the children enjoyed very much. In 1965, Ben and Estelle had a final marital disagreement. He offered to stay with her in Beverly Hills for six months of the year and then he would stay in France with his mistress for the other six months. She declined the arrangement and Ben Graham left Beverly Hills permanently.

Life in Beverly Hills

Not long after the Sarnats had moved into the house on Maple Drive, Another dog appeared on the scene. Rhoda purchased a breed of dog known as a Keeshond from a special breeder. The puppy selected from the litter seemed to be the most aggressive and alert of all of them. He was a beautiful puppy and Rhoda named him Gunner. It was a Dutch breed and because of the heavy fur, they could hide guns on their bodies and serve as gunrunners during some of the Dutch wars. He looked like a small version of a German shepherd, about 18 inches high, was pretty, feisty, bright, alert and stubborn. Rhoda took him to training school but he proved to be incorrigible and, could not be trained. He would escape from the patio and run across the street to the Luella Parsons residence and relieve himself at her front door. Another incident that occurred that led Bernie to finally give him the boot was that on one Sunday, a leaking faucet in the patio required calling a plumber who, in the process of making repairs, had disassembled the faucet only to find a part missing on re-assembly. Bernie noticed that Gunner seemed to be hiding something and sure enough it was that part. After chasing Gunner all aver the patio, Bernie finally retrieved the part. But this event was the proverbial one that "broke the camel's back" and Gunner had to go. They offered to give this pure breed and expensive dog away and no one would accept him. Finally, they approached the breeder and he agreed to take him back. Bernie and Rhoda were much relieved. In 1961, Jenny, a wonderful poodle entered their lives.

Mother Gerard, who lived about eight miles from the Sarnats, from the time she moved to California in 1955 until she died in 1963, would come over for dinner every Tuesday night. As she did not drive, she had to be picked up and dropped off. On Sundays the Sarnats would visit her at her apartment and then the five of them would go out for dinner. When Gerry became old enough to drive he took on the responsibility of picking her up and driving her home on Tuesdays and Sundays.

From 1963 on until both Gerry and Joan had married, Gerry in 1969 and Joan in 1975, both children had been attending college. When they returned from college at Christmas vacation, the four Sarnats would go out to dinner at a favorite English pub, the Cock and Bull on Sunset Boulevard. This was a charming, comfortable, cozy place with a warm atmosphere. The Sarnats had many fond memories of dinners there. Another fine restaurant on Sunset Boulevard was Scandia. Neither of these restaurants is in existence today. Also of slightly lesser quality, was Frascati, a Belgian restaurant chain that is, unfortunately also gone.

Life in Los Angeles

With Gerry married and gone, and Joan at the University of Michigan, Bernie and Rhoda no longer felt the need to keep up a large home. So in May of 1972, after selling the home, they had one final party for all of their friends; that is, a "house cooling," after which they moved into a very lovely apartment on Holmby Avenue in West Los Angeles, where they no longer planned to entertain large groups. In addition, there was no longer a need for full-time help since Rhoda was now busy as a faculty member in the School of Social Work at the University of Southern California. However, they were so devoted to Emma that they did keep her in their employ. It was now relatively easy for her to take care of the apartment and walk the poodle, Jenny. She came four days a week and left after dinner. In 1975, Emma died of a carcinoma of the breast. The Sarnats had lost a very faithful and devoted member of the family. In 1980, the Sarnats bought a more suitable condominium on Kelton Avenue, several blocks away from their earlier apartment on Holmby Avenue. They have been living here for over two decades and are extremely happy with their condominium.

As they have grown older, they have lost friends along the way and their social circle has shrunk considerably. As a result they have been doing much less entertaining. However, in 1985, Bernie organized a birthday party for Rhoda for her 70th birthday which he held at the Century Plaza Hotel, Beverly Hills. In 1991, for their 50th wedding anniversary, Bernie and Rhoda took the entire family on a cruise to Mexico for about 10 days (Fig. 24). On August 28th 1992, for Bernie's 80th birthday, they held a boat party at Marina del Rey for a number of their very close friends and families.

On September 10, 2005 Gerry and Joan had a 90th birthday party for Rhoda as well as a 60th birthday party for Gerry at the Boulevard Restaurant in San Francisco. The entire Sarnat family of 13 were present as well as other immediate members of the family, totaling about 25 people. They enjoyed the evening where Bernie showed slides of Rhoda, from few months old to the present. In addition, Joan arranged a song for the occasion and Gerry gave some wonderful introductory remarks (Fig. 53).

Of course while Gerry and Joan were home before going off to college, the four Sarnats took a number of trips together (Fig. 23 and Fig. 25). San Diego was a favorite place to visit because of the San Diego Zoo, the Wild Animal Park, and Sea World. In addition, visits to Catalina Island, Disneyland and some of the state parks, in particular Yosemite, were frequent places, while Santa Barbara, Solvang and Ojai were other favorite spots (Fig. 26). The next chapter relates Bernie and Rhoda's international travel.

Chapter **26**

FOREIGN TRAVEL

In 1961 Bernie and Rhoda planned an extensive trip to Europe. This would be his first while Rhoda, of course, had spent two years there earlier in her youth. Since the contemplated trip was going to be quite extensive, Bernie had a complete physical examination in April of that year. At that time he had a sigmoidoscopy done. This was a rigid sigmoidoscope placed internally into the rectum about 20 cm. It showed that everything was normal. Bernie found that he had a hernia at this time so he had the hernia and hemorrhoids repaired at the same time. After this he was told that he was in perfect health and ready to take on the vigorous trip to Europe.

The trip was sponsored by the Los Angeles County Medical Society as a trip for physicians and their spouses. This was in 1961 and the transition from propeller-driven aircraft to jet propulsion was not yet complete. So their trip was solely on a propeller-driven plane which necessitated frequent stops. They attempted to have the flight changed to a jet, which would have greatly shortened the flight time, but that was not feasible. The tour director tried to show them as much of Europe in the thirty-three days as possible. As a result, most of the stops were of one or two day's duration and at most three days. The countries that were visited included England, Belgium, Netherlands, France, Germany, Switzerland and Italy. The tour started and ended in France. It was a very rigorous journey. Toward the end of the trip they were in Nice, where they visited some of Rhoda's old haunts. Rhoda wanted to show Bernie where she had lived as a young girl in 1928. It was a bit of a walk from their hotel to the apartment where she had lived on the Promenade des Anglais. They were also able to gain access to the tenants who were then living in the apartment. After walking back from her apartment to their hotel, Bernie experienced severe exhaustion and attributed this to fatigue from the rather rigorous trip they were on. It turned out that this fatigue was the start of life threatening consequences, which affected his surgical practice as well his life for a number of years (see Chapter 27 for details).

By 1964, Bernie had returned to a full-time normal program. He had been invited to speak in Israel as well as Denmark and London. With Rhoda, he arranged the trip first to Israel where he spoke at Hebrew University and also at Tel Aviv University, again visiting in 1994 (Fig. 47). From there they went to Denmark where he spoke at the Royal Dental College in Copenhagen. The Sarnats were hosted by Dr. Arne Björk, who was head of the department of orthodontics and had an international reputation for his work on facial growth. While visiting the laboratories, Bernie met Dr. Gordon Nikiforuk whom he had known at the University of Illinois in the late 1930's. Dr. Nikiforuk told Bernie that he would be soon joining him in Los Angeles at the newly formed dental school at UCLA. He eventually became Head of Oral Biology and Associate Dean at UCLA and later left to return to the University of Toronto Dental School as Dean. After touring Copenhagen, Rhoda and Bernie then went on to England. After several days in England, Bernie spoke at Guy's Hospital, having been invited by Dr. Ronald Emsley. This proved to be a highly successful trip and Bernie experienced no difficulties whatsoever from his cancer surgery and chemotherapy (see Chapter 27).

Another extensive trip that Bernie and Rhoda took was to Japan and Hong Kong in November of 1966. This trip was sponsored by the Los Angeles County Art Museum. While in Tokyo, word was received that Ronald Reagan had defeated the incumbent Pat Brown for governor of California. This trip to Japan proved to be a wonderful experience in travel.

Soon after they had returned from Japan, Bernie received a call at his office from their former housekeeper, Emma, whom they had engaged in Chicago from 1947 to 1955. She indicated that she and her husband had decided to move to California. Bernie did not tell Rhoda, Gerry or Joan. She came over the next afternoon when the family was home and they were indeed happily surprised when she met them all at the front door. Bernie had invited her to come to the 25th wedding anniversary party. Bernie asked her if she would like to come back to the family as housekeeper. She readily agreed and once again became the housekeeper for the Sarnats.

Bernie and Rhoda made plans to hold their 25th wedding anniversary party. When Bernie was ill with cancer in 1961, relatives and friends visited him in Madison, Wisconsin to offer their encouragement, where he was receiving chemotherapy. He had promised that if he were still alive in 1966 he would have an outstanding 25th wedding anniversary party to which they would all be invited. In late December 1966, family and friends gathered at 616 North Maple Drive. Friends came from the Chicago area, New Haven, Connecticut, Irvine, California, Los Angeles and Beverly Hills. They attended a cocktail party and a sit down dinner. The living room and the adjoining music room were spacious enough for the 65 guests for the formal dinner (Figs. 18 to 22).

Bernie's brother-in-law Leo Spira acted as the master of ceremonies for the evening. There was much singing and reminiscing and two skits that proved to be the highlights at the end of the evening. One was by Gerry and Joan who were back from the East Coast for the Christmas break. Rhoda had been sharing Bernie's office where he was seeing his patients for surgery and she was also seeing her patients for psychotherapy. The basis of the skit by Gerry and Joan was that these patients were inadvertently mixed up in that Bernie had Rhoda's patients and Rhoda had Bernie's patients. The skit proved to be quite hilarious. The last and final event of the evening was a song, Sunrise and Sunset from Fiddler on the Roof, sung by Joan and her high school boyfriend, Jon. Jon played the guitar to accompany their singing. This proved to be the stellar event of the evening that "brought down the house." As a memento of the occasion each guest received a specially selected Kennedy half-dollar encased in a custom prepared plastic case.

By 1966 Bernie and the family had settled down and were now pretty much leading a normal routine. They would be entertaining at home. Some would be small dinner parties of about 10 or 12 people and the evenings to be spent in discussions of various topics. A few large cocktail parties were held outdoors in the patio and garden for as many as 100 people. Because of the size of the grounds there was no problem accommodating numbers of this size.

Bernie presented a paper on rabbit snout growth at the 4th International Congress of Plastic Surgeons in Rome, Italy.[1] At that meeting Paul Tessier from Paris presented his outstanding work which opened up the new field of craniofacial surgery (Fig. 31). Bernie then flew to Lisbon and met Rhoda on Friday, October 13, 1967. They toured Portugal and Spain for about four weeks.

Living continued along quite smoothly and in 1969, they planned a trip to East Africa and South Africa under the auspices of the Los Angeles Zoo. The tour group included about 30 individuals, many members of the Los Angeles Zoo. Bernie and Rhoda shared the trip in particular with Irving and Jean Stone. While in Johannesburg, the group attended a cocktail party with some of the local residents. For Bernie, they invited several physicians. When he told them during the conversation that he would be at dinner with a young physician who wanted to study plastic surgery in the United States, they immediately responded by saying that he must be either British or Jewish. Bernie was quite surprised by the statement. He later learned that these were "Dutch" or Afrikaner doctors who would never leave the country for overseas study.

While in Johannesburg, Bernie and Rhoda attended a dinner given by the chief of pediatric surgery who was Jewish. There they met his son who was interested in becoming a plastic surgeon. Bernie gave his best advice and he subsequently ended up as a prominent plastic surgeon in Cleveland, Ohio.

From Johannesburg they flew to Cape Town where Rhoda had a cousin, Roma Harris, who had lived there for many years and the last time she had seen her was at the family reunion in Vichy, France in 1928. Following this, for about three weeks, they traveled on safari to the various national parks to view and photograph the animals in their natural settings. The trip ended in Nairobi. There, they were invited to dinner at the home of one of their tour guides, John Williams, originally from England, who was an outstanding ornithologist. Interestingly, before they left for Africa, Rhoda had gone to a bookstore in Beverly Hills and purchased a book on the Birds of Africa. The author was none other than the John Williams who turned out to be one of their guides. His English wife was a physician who at that time was trying to introduce birth-control to a segment of the Nairobi population. Her project was fraught with problems and ended unsuccessfully.

Their other guide, also an Englishman, was Colonel Cowie, a former British military man, immaculately groomed with a beautiful, well trimmed full mustache. He was the expert on four-legged animals.

During the safari, most of the time was spent in accommodations that were tents. Toward the end of the safari, the group was treated to a most unusual experience. They spent the day and night at William Holden's most delightful rendezvous. The grounds were spacious and well groomed with a wide variety of plants, flowers and trees. Tame birds were wandering on the grounds. The Sarnats and Stones shared a beautiful log cabin. An attendant took care of the fireplace with logs and turned their bed covers down. The European cuisine was superb. The chef was from Europe. It was a most wonderful and unexpected experience in the heart of East Africa.

From Nairobi the group flew to Rome and there the Sarnats spent three full days with the Stones. Irving and Jean had spent two years in Rome researching material for the highly popular book: *The Agony and the Ecstasy*. They enjoyed taking Bernie and Rhoda around to their favorite haunts. It was a wonderful way to culminate an outstanding trip (Fig. 33 and Fig. 34).

Over the ensuing years, Bernie and Rhoda traveled extensively in the United States and Canada including Alaska and Hawaii. This included a seven-day rafting trip down the Colorado River, traveling to the North and South Rims, flying over the Grand Canyon, and a donkey trek up from the bottom of the Grand Canyon.

Their travels also took them to Mexico, Guatemala, and Ecuador with the Galapagos Islands, Machu Picchu, Peru, Amazon basin and Brazil (Figs. 37 to 39). Of course they traveled to England, France, Switzerland and Italy several times. In addition, they went to Denmark, Finland, Norway, Sweden, Belgium, the Netherlands, Austria, Monaco, Yugoslavia, Gibraltar, Greece and the Greek islands, Egypt, Turkey and Israel. They were also in the USSR, along the Volga River, India, Sri Lanka, Nepal (Fig. 41), Pakistan, the Kashmir, Vietnam, Thailand, Philippines, Taiwan, Australia and New Zealand. One memorable trip took Bernie to China (Fig. 35 and Fig. 36). Also involved were cruises to the Eastern Mediterranean, on the Danube River, the Eastern and Western Caribbean, Alaska, Canada, Saint Lawrence River, and Panama Canal. On all of these trips Rhoda would be equipped with the latest Minolta camera and various lenses. She was quite a photography buff.

The last trip that Rhoda and Bernie took abroad was to France in 1989. This trip was in part initiated because David, Joan's husband, had a six-month visiting professorship at the University of Paris. Joan's family lived there while their two boys went to school. After visiting with them, Bernie and Rhoda toured northern France before returning to the States.

Chapter 27

A CLOSE BRUSH WITH DEATH

As related in the last chapter, while on their travels to Nice, France, Bernie experienced severe tiredness and attributed this largely to the stresses related to the rather rigorous European trip. Their return to Los Angeles and Beverly Hills in June 1961 from the trip abroad was uneventful and Bernie went back into his normal routine, professionally and personally. On July 24th, he came home for lunch and had an ear of corn. That evening they were invited out to dinner and again had corn-on-the-cob, which they enjoyed. During the night he suffered from a bowel obstruction. A barium enema was done and it was found that it could not pass the obstructed site. A tentative diagnosis was made of carcinoma of the sigmoid bowel. The sigmoidoscopy that had been conducted a few months earlier had stopped just short of the region of the bowel that was involved with the carcinoma. Before going in for surgery early that morning, Bernie awakened Gerry to tell him that he was going into the hospital to be operated on and was in serious trouble. He told Gerry that he would now have to help Rhoda to become head of the household and share some of the responsibilities. This was a great burden to put on a young son of about 16.

Cancer of the Bowel: Surgery

A bowel resection was done the next day by his very good surgical friend, Nathan Barshop, and some twelve regional lymph nodes were found to contain metastases. Fortunately, no metastases where found in the liver. After five hours' of surgery, Bernie was returned to his room. When the surgeon came up afterward, Rhoda said that he looked worse than Bernie did. The next day after the surgery, Bernie reviewed the pathology slides with his good friend, Leo Kaplan, the pathologist. He then put the question directly to the pathologist as to the prognosis. His friend shook his head and said six months. With this discouraging information, the next day Bernie was on the telephone, both locally and nationally, seeking further advice. He was advised, fortunately, not to have radiation therapy. But in a book that Bernie had written on oral and facial cancer, Paul Kotin had contributed a chapter. Dr. Kotin had spent a year in the oncology department at the University of Wisconsin in Madison. This was where the chemotherapy drug 5FUDR (5-fluorouracildeoxyriboflavin) had been developed for the treatment of cancer of the bowel. He assured Bernie that he would walk in and would walk out. In the past, patients at that time receiving 5FU in Los Angeles would generally die because of the toxicity of the drug and also the advanced stage of the disease.

On the ninth postoperative day, Bernie flew to Madison, Wisconsin. The following day he was started on 5FUDR, a modification of 5FU. Rhoda joined him the next day since she had to take Joan to summer camp. Gerry stayed with friends and was enrolled in summer school. While Bernie and Rhoda were in Madison, they had a number of friends, relatives, colleagues and students visit them. Bernie had been instructed to eat a high protein diet and when some of his friends took him out to dinner and he would order roast beef, take one or two bites but because of the nausea from taking 5FUDR, he could not finish his dinner.

After about a week Bernie was sent home to Beverly Hills with the chemotherapy medication and continued the treatment given by his personal physician. Upon their return to Beverly Hills, several things happened. First, the news of Bernie's problem had spread far and wide, locally, nationally and internationally. He was amazed at how fast word had spread and how many had already assumed his demise. Upon Bernie's return to Beverly Hills, he continued his chemotherapy. Although the effects were quite severe, including nausea and oral ulcerations, he managed to continue, in a limited way, ordinary living and a limited amount of his private practice. With all his problems, Bernie and Rhoda decided that they better pick cemetery plots, which they did. It also had an effect on his private practice, so he arranged to meet with George Cordingly, the owner of the office building where Bernie had just signed a five-year lease a few months before. Upon presentation of this problem, Cordingly spontaneously offered that as long as Bernie was not able to work full time the rent could be reduced by 50%. This helped Bernie's spirits considerably.

Rhoda and Bernie also discussed the possible sale of their lovely home at 616 North Maple Drive which in the event of Bernie's death, Rhoda would probably no longer be able to support and the family could no longer afford to live there. The general consensus was that the home be sold and the family move into an apartment. After much discussion between them and with a close friend, a real-tor, who advised them not to do anything but to just "sit tight." This is what they did and it proved to be good advice.[1]

By now the home had been completely furnished and Rhoda had time for other activities. Within two to three weeks after Rhoda and Bernie's return to Beverly Hills, Rhoda came home one day with a young poodle puppy, called Jenny, and who, to everybody's delight, proved to be a wonderful dog. Jenny eventually had four puppies at one time and lived to be about 16 years old. She proved to be an invaluable member of the family during a very difficult period.

Bernie during this time was also in touch with several physicians nationally and learned that for a carcinoma of the bowel, a second look was suggested about six to 10 months after the surgery. Dr. Wangensteen at the University of Minnesota School of medicine was an advocate of this and Bernie was in touch with him. He finally suggested that Bernie have this done about eight months after the initial surgery. Bernie had known him previously having participated in one of the programs Dr. Wangensteen had produced.

Thus, in May of 1962 he returned to Chicago for a "second look." The reason that Bernie went to Chicago was that a very experienced surgeon, Dr. Pete Rosi, who would do the radical surgery was there. One purpose was to check to see if it had spread to the liver and elsewhere. When he saw Dr. Rosi in his office the day before the exploratory surgery, Bernie said: "that if the cancer had spread to the liver that he was to do radical surgery and take it out." At that time, liver surgery was in its infancy. When Bernie recovered from the anesthesia the day after surgery, Dr. Rosi told him that he had taken 14 biopsies and on both the gross inspection and microscopic examination of tissue had not found any cancer in any of the biopsies nor in the liver or anywhere else for that matter. Wonder of wonders! Who could have expected such an uplifting report? With this news life began anew, for the Sarnats. It is now more than 46 years since the surgery with no recurrence. Because of the unusualness of the postoperative recovery, the details of Bernie's rather rare carcinoma were eventually published in a medical journal.[2]

A Successful Recovery

Bernie and Rhoda were superbly overjoyed to receive such unexpectedly good news. The family and friends who had visited Bernie during this time were also very happy and Bernie said that if after five years, which was known as a "five-year cure," a time which would coincide with their 25th wedding anniversary, he would hold a big party for everyone if he was still around. A discussion of this party is in Chapter 26.

They then returned to Los Angeles and although Bernie was convinced that he might be cured, he was still concerned that microscopic remains might have been mobilized due to the manipulations during the exploratory surgery. To dispel his fears, Bernie convinced the physicians at the University of Wisconsin to send him a fourth course of treatment. He withstood that satisfactorily and at no time did he ever have a loss of hair although soreness of the mouth was a frequent problem. For a period of about two years, Bernie tried to lead a somewhat normal but restricted life. He limited his surgical practice as well.

Finally, it was mentioned earlier that while in Chicago in 1956, Bernie had noticed blood in his stool and called his very good friend and internist, Seymour Weisberg, who immediately examined him and diagnosed that he had a hemorrhoid. But Bernie, who at that time was still not that far removed from his medical training, insisted on a second opinion. This led to another friend, Mort Baker, who was a very capable radiologist, who did a barium enema at Bernie's request and found that the findings were normal. Bernie took those X-ray films with him and in 1961 after the surgery for the CA of the bowel, those films were reviewed and they found that in one area where the carcinoma was excised in 1961, there was a polyp. So in hindsight it was felt that the initial examination should have been repeated to check more closely to see whether that polyp could have given rise to the carcinoma.

Chapter 28

PRIVATE PRACTICE IN BEVERLY HILLS (1956–1991)

Bernie's practice of plastic and reconstructive surgery in Chicago required considerable driving. His office was in the downtown region on South Michigan Boulevard and the hospitals that he used were scattered from the Westside to the far Southside of Chicago. In addition, he had responsibilities at the University of Illinois while he lived on the Southside. So, in the course of the day he would drive anywhere from 20 to 30 miles. All of the driving was made more difficult with the cold weather, ice, and snow in the wintertime.

Bernie was determined that moving to California would hopefully make the driving less extensive and less difficult. The moderate climate of Los Angeles and Beverly Hills was a great improvement. Once settled, he began to also look for an office there. Through a friend of Bernie's in Chicago, he met a doctor, Jesse Garber who was about to open a new office at 435 North Roxbury Drive in Beverly Hills. This office was ideal for two physicians to practice in. This was in a medical triangle bounded by Camden Drive, Santa Monica Boulevard and Wilshire Boulevard. In this several block area was an extremely well qualified medical community of some 400 medical specialists.

Bernie was the fourth American Board of Plastic Surgery specialist in Beverly Hills (Today there are over 50 such specialists).

Coincidentally, he learned that the Garber family from New York knew Rhoda's cousin, Ben Graham, very well. In addition, Rhoda's mother and Jesse Garber's mother had been friends in New York. His next problem was to obtain hospital privileges. Just adjacent to Beverly Hills on the Eastern side, a new hospital, Mount Sinai, had been opened about one year. There were a number of applicants at the hospital, which also had a long waiting list for appointments to the medical staff. Because Bernie had come with not only a national but also an international reputation, he was given top priority and within two months received an appointment. So now quite in contrast to Chicago, he had his home, office, and hospital appointment all within a one-mile radius. Several miles to the east was another rather excellent hospital, Cedars of Lebanon, where he soon received an appointment. In that same region was Temple Hospital where he was able to get an immediate appointment.

Having taken the medical state board in California in 1937, Bernie had no difficulty in re-activating his medical license. Subsequently, he also obtained staff privileges at Beverly Hills Doctors Hospital where he did most of his aesthetic surgery. The difficult cases in plastic and reconstructive surgery were generally done at Mount Sinai and Cedars of Lebanon Hospitals. In 1968, the medical staffs of Cedars of Lebanon Hospital and Mount Sinai Hospital merged. In 1976, the new, extremely well-equipped, modern thousand-bed Cedars-Sinai Hospital opened on the Mount Sinai Hospital grounds. Bernie served as Chief of Plastic Surgery for over 20 years at these hospitals, both before and after they merged.

In 1980, the Bernard G. Sarnat, M.D. Annual Lectureship in Plastic Surgery was established at the Cedars-Sinai Medical Center.

In about 1958, because there were very few well-trained plastic surgeons in the San Fernando Valley, a region north of Beverly Hills, Bernie opened a second office at 4849 Van Nuys Boulevard. He maintained it for several years, sharing office space with a former University of Chicago medical classmate, Dr. Edward Cantor.

By the end of the five-year lease at the Beverly Hills office, Dr. Garber had decided to move to a new office. Bernie agreed to take over the office and signed a new five-year lease. Five months later, as described in Chapter 27, Bernie was operated on for cancer of the bowel.

Now that Bernie had established where to live, practice, and the necessary hospital affiliations, it remained for him to make himself known in the community at large. With his reputation established, he was invited to speak before various medical and dental societies, schools and hospitals staffs. He was very busy in the first year or two, lecturing quite frequently. Of course, some patients continued to come to him from a national and even international referral. By the end of the first year, Bernie's income had more than offset his expenses.

Bernie had been trained to treat patients with burns, hand problems, and neck tumors. These surgical problems had become more specialized. Consequently, by mid-1960's he had stopped doing these surgeries. Also, his practice had never quite recovered from the shock of his illness in 1961. By 1980, Bernie was 68 years old and decided to begin limiting his practice further. He sublet office space at 9735 Wilshire Boulevard until November 21, 1991, his last day, when he retired from the practice of plastic and reconstructive surgery. He transferred his practice and records to Dr. Robin Yuan on November 22, 1991, a Harvard Medical School graduate who was board certified in both general and plastic surgery.

Bernie, however, continued that part of his life that had been devoted to academic pursuits such as research, teaching and writing as a Senior Research Scientist at Cedars-Sinai Medical Center and as Adjunct Professor of Oral Biology, School of Dentistry and Plastic Surgery, School of Medicine at UCLA.

Bernie had a number of prominent patients known locally, nationally and internationally from the business and entertainment professions. Because of privacy concerns no names will be mentioned.

The almost fifty years of practice in plastic and reconstructive surgery (1943–1991) were most gratifying years. During this time Bernie did the usual aesthetic surgery such as facelifts, eye plastics, cleft lip and palates, tumors of the face and jaws, nasal plastics, breast reductions and up-lifts, abdominoplasties, skin grafting and a variety of other conditions. Nevertheless, four patients in particular stand out and have remained in his mind through the years.

Patient #1: Cleft lip and palate

This patient was born with a complete cleft lip and palate. Bernie knew what the parents were in for and had to prepare himself before talking with them as to what the future held, not only for the child in the surgical repair and emotional trauma, but also the problems that the parents would have to face as well. It was not an unusually difficult case and the surgical results were quite satisfactory. Nevertheless, there was a scar of the lip, some deformity of the nose and some speech difficulty as well. As the infant grew, all these problems were faced and treated in due time. The mother, a social worker, and the father an attorney, were both well-informed individuals but as time passed they had difficulty adjusting to the problems that they encountered with their child. Regrettably, although these two people were very intelligent parents and had had joint counseling, apparently the birth of a child with a deformity was enough to result in a divorce. The child remained with the mother who raised her to become relatively normal when last seen at about ten years of age.

Patient #2: Battered Infant Syndrome

Bernie was called into the emergency room at Cedars of Lebanon Hospital in Los Angeles to see a six week-old infant who had a possible fractured mandible. The father, who had brought the child in, said that he had the infant lying on a couch when he walked into the other room and when he came back the infant had rolled off the couch onto the floor. Bernie, observing the child, saw that there were black and blue marks, which were not of recent origin. X-ray pictures taken of the mandible displayed two fractures, which was most unusual for a six-week old infant. Because the story did not seem tenable, upon further questioning, the father admitted that both he and his wife had been beating the infant over the last several days because it was crying. Because this was a criminal offense, the Department of Social Services was called in and the child was made a ward of the court. The father was jailed and the mother placed in the Sybil Brand Institute, a women's facility. Because of the abuse, further medical workup was necessary and permission had to be obtained from the court.

Concern about brain damage and other trauma required a spinal puncture for blood and an examination of the abdominal fluid for blood to rule out a possible ruptured internal organ as well as additional x-ray pictures of various regions. The only significant injuries were the two fractures of the mandible. Treatment of the edentulous mandible in a six-week old infant required considerable planning and imagination. The infant became very popular in the pediatric division of the hospital and was eventually placed in a foster home.

Patient #3: De Cubitus Ulcer of the Buttock

A 56 year-old woman had been found lying on her back, unconscious in her room where she lived alone. She had probably been this way for several days. By lying on her back the pressure of the pelvis on the soft tissues had created a large ulcer, a result of the bony pressure on soft tissues obstructing the blood supply. She was brought to the hospital, having regained consciousness. The wound was cleansed and the necrotic tissue trimmed. A thick amount of tissue, a flap of local tissue, was then rotated in to cover the bony prominence of the ischial tuberosity of the pelvis. After the surgical procedure the patient was able to ambulate normally.

Patient #4: Dog Bite of Nose

It was the 4th of July at an outdoor barbecue. A family was having a number of guests to celebrate the holiday and the host was barbecuing. Their German shepherd, a member of the family for several years, who had been a wonderful dog, quite suddenly jumped up and bit off the tip of her nose. End of barbecue. Fortunately, the tip of the nose was recovered and placed in chipped ice. The patient was then seen in the emergency room at Cedars of Lebanon Hospital. To the patient's and the surgeon's pleasant surprise, the surgery proved to be successful.

Finally, to conclude this chapter on a lighter note, in Bernie's talks to the non-plastic surgical profession about plastic surgery, there were two "stories" that he liked to pass on to the audience.

A Mrs. Goldberg had brought her daughter in for a nasal plastic procedure. This 15-year-old attractive and personable young lady had a typical hump of the nose. About the seventh day after the surgical procedure, Doctor Sarnat called Mrs. Goldberg into the examining room to see the result. As she shifted from one foot to the other, Bernie knew that a question would be forthcoming. She asked: "Dr. Sarnat when my daughter gets married and has children would her children have noses like my daughter's before the operation or after the operation?" Bernie waited for a moment and being a biologist as he likes to think he is, said "Mrs. Goldberg they have been circumcising Jewish boys for thousands of years and they still have to be circumcised."

Another story that Bernie liked to tell was about a surgical procedure, a general body lift. A 70-year-old man came into the office with loose skin of the face, the chin, the neck, the arms, the chest, the abdomen, the thighs and legs, etc. The patient said: "Dr. Sarnat can you help me?" The doctor responded by saying: "Of course" He then stepped up on a stool and lifted the patient up by the scalp and all the loose tissue of the face, chin, neck, arms, chest etc., came up to the scalp. He then placed a tie at the base of the excess tissue and cut it off. The patient returned one week later and Bernie asked him how he liked the results. The patient replied: "Great, but I never had a dimple in my chin before." Bernie responded by saying: "think nothing of it, that is your belly button, and by the way what do you think of the jazzy bow-tie I gave you?"

Chapter 29

ACADEMIA AND RESEARCH (1956–PRESENT)

A fter Bernie had determined that his family was adequately set-tled down and his private practice of plastic and reconstructive surgery was developing nicely, he turned his attention to academia and research.

Academia

Soon after Bernie arrived in Los Angeles he was approached by the Dean of the University of Southern California Dental School, Robert McNulty. Bernie had known him in Chicago when he was Associate Dean at the Chicago College of Dental Surgery, Loyola University. Dr. McNulty offered him a position in the Department of Oral Surgery which did not interest him very much because he did not consider himself as an oral surgeon. He wanted to continue his practice in plastic and reconstructive surgery. In addition, since at that time basic research did not have a high priority at the Dental School, he did not accept the offer.

Since the University of Southern California, School of Medicine, Division of Plastic and Reconstructive Surgery was not very well developed, it also did not sound promising. In addition, since Bernie lived on the Westside of Los Angeles, this added the considerable burden of driving to the Eastern part of Los Angeles, which was not a great inducement for Bernie.

261

At the University of California at Los Angeles (UCLA) which was on the Westside of Los Angeles and adjacent to where Bernie lived, a fledgling medical school had just been founded in the 1950's. The Medical School was still housed in Quonset huts. The first class of medical students was graduated in 1955. Sometime in the 1960's, Franklin Ashley had been appointed acting Chief of the Division of Plastic and Reconstructive Surgery. Soon thereafter, Ashley offered Bernie an appointment which he refused because of personal differences. Several years later, Harvey Zarem was appointed as the first full-time Chief of Plastic and Reconstructive Surgery at UCLA. He offered Bernie an appointment which he immediately accepted. The appointment as full-professor was officially recognized in 1974 by the university. Bernie continues to be active in the Division of Plastic and Reconstructive Surgery and his appointment is at the highest professorial level.

Prior to the 1960's there was no dental school at UCLA. In the early 1960's, the California State Legislature appropriated funds for such a dental school. Bernie had been invited to a number of dinner meetings exploring the needs of the future dental school. At one of those meetings it had been proposed that the Dental School be built on Veterans Administration grounds several blocks away from the proposed new permanent Medical School buildings. Bernie vigorously opposed this concept and stressed that the new Dental School building should be in close proximity to the new Medical School buildings, a situation that became reality. He was eventually offered a full professorship in the Department of Oral and Maxillofacial Surgery in the Dental School, which he refused. The reason for the refusal being that his primary interest was in continuing his basic research. He requested an appointment in the Section of Oral Biology. This appointment was eventually formalized in 1967 and Bernie has taught continuously there since the first class entered the Dental School in 1967.

Research

By now Bernie had renewed his focus on research. He had brought a great deal of material from the University of Illinois which required further organization and preparation. These spanned the years 1956 to 1960 and led to numerous publications. Fortunately, he was able to transfer his NIH grant[1-6] from the University of Illinois to California.

Additionally, a big plus for Bernie was his clinical appointment (Chap. 28) at Cedars of Lebanon Hospital where there was a research institute. Research initiated there resulted in a number of publications during the period 1961 to 1971 and later.[7-20] Subsequently, Bernie transferred his laboratory from Cedars of Lebanon, located at that time near Vermont Ave. and Sunset Blvd., to the new Mount Sinai research Institute at Beverly Blvd. and San Vicente Ave., and during the period 1963 to 1998 there were numerous additional publications.[21-36] Moreover, this move was much closer to where he lived and where his office was located. Later, Bernie transferred his laboratory facilities, to the UCLA Dental Research Institute and the School of Medicine in Westwood. Research done there with undergraduate and graduate students as well as faculty, resulted in a number of publications spanning the years 1968 to 1995.[37-46]

In conjunction with Andrew Dixon, former Dean of the Dental School, Bernie jointly organized three international congresses on bone biology (Fig. 40). More than 15 disciplines and 15 different countries were represented at these three congresses in 1982, 1985, and 2000.[47-49] A volume of each meeting was published. In addition, the third (1980)[50] and fourth (1991)[51] editions of the widely used text: *The Temporomandibular Joint: Basic Science and Clinical Practice* was published. This book was also translated into Japanese and published in Japan (1983).[52] The textbook *Oral Facial Cancers* had a second edition published in 1958 and was translated into Portuguese and published in Brazil (1956).[53]

Scientific Contributions

One can summarize Bernie's considerable scientific contributions as follows: (1) he was a prime contributor to the fundamental knowledge and the early foundation of the specialty of craniofacial biology; (2) he was the first to display the presence of phosphorus bands in the base of the skull at the spheno-occipital and spheno-ethmoidal synchondroses[54]; (3) he was able to demonstrate the important role that vital stains and radio-opaque implants play determining the growth of bones and teeth[55-60]; (4) he was the first to quantitatively measure the deceleration effects of hibernation on growth of dentin with use of vital stains[61]; (5) he was also among the first to determine the effect of experimental surgical procedures on bone growth[54,55,62-64]; (6) he conducted extensive studies on the nature of sutural, appositional and resorptive bone growth[65]; (7) he also made other fundamental contributions to bone growth; (8) he was the first to use tritiated thymidine to study the growth of the cartilaginous nasal septum[66]; (9) he was the initial investigator to develop the use of orbital imprints[67]; (10) he was the first to demonstrate that an underlying membrane was not essential for the re-growth of a suture[68]; (11) his report on the growth pattern of the nasal bone was probably the first[69]; and (12) he demonstrated the appearance of severe facial deformity produced by resection of the cartilaginous nasal septum in young rabbits.[70]

In 1984, the Bernard G. Sarnat International Lectureship in Bone Biology was established at UCLA as a forum to bring in worldwide specialists in bone biology to present their research. This successful program is now in its 22nd year and is widely attended by students and faculty in Medicine and Dentistry (Table 5).

Clinical Contributions

His clinical contributions are also noteworthy and can be listed as: (1) he demonstrated the important role of teeth as recorders of systemic disease[71,72]; (2) he also confirmed radiographically the early findings in congenital syphilis of un-erupted permanent teeth[73,74]; (3) he also established over a 16-year study period that teeth do not play a role in the growth of the jaws except for alveolar bone[75]; (4) he was the first to describe the x-ray findings of the jaws in

Table 5. Bernard G. Sarnat International Lectureship in Bone Biology, UCLA School of Dentistry.

1	Paul Tessier, M.D. Foch Hospital, Päris, France	1984
2	Per Ingvar Branemark, M.D., Ph.D. University of Göteborg, Sweden	1985
3	David L. Rimoin, M.D., Ph.D. Cedars-Sinai Medical Center, Los Angeles, USA	1986
4	David A. N. Hoyte, M.D., MRCGP, University of Nottingham, England	1988
5	David E. Poswillo, D.D.S., D.Sc., M.D. University of London, England	1989
6	M. Michael Cohen, Jr., D.M.D., Ph.D. Dalhousie University, Halifax, Nova Scotia	1990
7	Melvin J. Glimcher, M.D. Harvard Medical School, Boston, USA	1991
8	David J. Baylink, M.D. Loma Linda University, Loma Linda, USA	1992
9	N. Scott Adzick, M.D. UCSF School of Medicine, San Francisco, USA	1993
10	Brian K. Hall, Ph.D., D.Sc., FRSC Dalhousie University, Halifax, Nova Scotia	1994
11	Raymond L. Hintz, M.D. Stanford University, Palo Alto, USA	1995
12	Joseph G. McCarthy, M.D. New York University Medical Center, USA	1996
13	Robert J. Gorlin, D.D.S., D.Sc. University of Minnesota, USA	1997
14	Harold C. Slavkin, D.D.S. NIDCR, Bethesda, M.D., USA	1998
15	Bernard G. Sarnat, M.D., D.D.S. University of California, Los Angeles, USA	1999
16	Donald H. Enlow, Ph.D. University of North Carolina, Chapel Hill, USA	2000
17	John M. Wozney, Ph.D. Genetics Institute Inc., Andover, MA, USA	2001
18	A. Hari Reddi, Ph.D. University of California, Davis, USA	2002
19	Susan Herring, Ph.D. University of Washington, Seattle, USA	2003
20	George W. Bernard, D.D.S., Ph.D. University of California, Los Angeles, USA	2004
21	Michael T. Longaker, M.D., FACS, Stanford University, Palo Alto, USA	2005
22	Geoffrey H. Sperber, Ph.D., FIDC, D.M.D. University of Alberta, Canada	2006
23	Jill Helms, D.D.S., Ph.D., Stanford University, Palo Alto, USA	2007

Table 6.   Bernard G. Sarnat Cedars-Sinai Lectureship.

1	Melvin Spira, M.D. Baylor University College of Medicine, Houston, TX	1980
2	Stephen J. Mathes, M.D. UCSF School of Medicine, San Francisco, CA	1983
3	John Bostwick III, M.D. Emory University School of Medicine, Atlanta, GA	1984
4	Foad Nahai, M.D. Emory University School of Medicine, Atlanta, GA	1986
5	John W. Little, M.D. Georgetown University, Washington, DC	1987
6	Ian I. Jackson, M.D., Mayo Clinic, Rochester, MN	1988
7	Joseph E. Murray*, M.D. Harvard Medical School, Boston, MA	1989
8	Malcom A. Lesavoy, M.D. UCLA School of Medicine, Los Angeles, CA	1990
9	Milton T. Edgerton, M.D. University of Virginia, Charlottesville, VA	1992
10	Jack Fisher, M.D. UCSF School of Medicine, San Francisco, CA	1993
11	Sam T. Hamra, M.D. University of Texas Health Science Center, Dallas, TX	1994
12	Rollin K. Daniel, M.D. UCI College of Medicine, Irvine, CA	1995
13	Jose Guerrerosantos, M.D. University of Guadalajara Medical School, Mexico	1996
14	John B. Tebbetts, M.D. University of Texas SW Medical School, Dallas, TX	1997
15	Gregory S. LaTrenta, M.D. Cornell University College of Medicine, New York	1998
16	James C. Grotting, M.D. University of Alabama at Birmingham, AL	1999
17	Robert S. Flowers, M.D. University of Hawaii School of Medicine, Honolulu	2000
18	Rodney J. Rohrich, M.D. University of Texas SW Medical School, Dallas, TX	2001
19	James M. Stuzin, M.D. University of Miami School of Medicine, Miami, FL	2001
20	Thomas R. Hester, M.D. Emory University School of Medicine, Atlanta, GA	2002
21	Foad Nahai, M.D. Emory University School of Medicine, Atlanta, GA	2002
22	David A. Hidalgo, M.D. Weill Medical College of Cornell University, Ithaca, NY	2003
23	Scott L. Spear, M.D. Georgetown University Hospital, Washington, DC	2004
24	Al S. Aly, M.D. Iowa City Plastic Surgery, Corlville, Iowa	2005
25	Jack Fisher, M.D. Vanderbilt University School of Medicine, Nashville, TN	2006
26	Glenn Jelks, M.D. New York, NY	2007

* Nobel Laureate in Physiology or Medicine, 1990.

sickle cell anemia[76]; (5) he recognized that yellow phosphorus added to cod liver oil given to children to develop more solid bone and prevent rickets, is a public health risk since it produces bone growth arrest[54]; (6) he published the first book on oral and facial cancer[77] which has been reprinted[78,79] and translated into foreign languages such as Portuguese[53]; and (7) he edited the first textbook correlating basic science with clinical practice in temporomandibular joint disorders.[80] It appeared in later editions[81,82,83] as well as translated into Japanese.[52]

In 1980, the Bernard G. Sarnat, M.D. Annual Lectureship in Plastic Surgery was established with Melvin Spira, M.D., as the first presenter at the Cedars-Sinai Medical Center. This lectureship, now in its 24th year, has been an outstanding success with the all-day meetings with more than 100 plastic surgeons in attendance. Speakers included internationally known figures such as Joseph Murray, M.D., a Nobel Laureate in Physiology or Medicine, 1990 (Fig. 44) (Table 6).

Chapter 30

A DAY IN THE LIFE OF A PLASTIC SURGEON

At the age of nine years, Bernie decided to become an oral and plastic surgeon. He was influenced by his 19-year-old brother who was a dental student. In medical school, he saw an occasional cleft lip and palate patient and a patient who had been burned. This was in the mid-1930's at a time when the specialty was young, growing and relatively undeveloped. As an intern, he was fortunate to be assigned to a combined oral surgery and ear, nose and throat program where he learned to treat facial trauma. As a dental student in the late 1930's, he treated an occasional fractured jaw, and in 1940 and 1941, he served as a resident in oral and plastic surgery. It was not until the mid-1940's however, when he spent three years with the famous Vilray P. Blair and Louis T. Byars in St. Louis, that Bernie became an accomplished general plastic and reconstructive surgeon. He learned to treat a wide variety of conditions over the whole body.

With this brief sketch of Bernie's early career, one might ask what a plastic surgeon's day is like.

(A) Reconstructive Surgery: Cleft Lip

Although treatment of this defect is reconstructive, there is a large and essential aesthetic component. During embryonic development in the human, at about five to six weeks of pregnancy, the right and left components of the upper lip occasionally fail to fuse. There can be just a slight notch of the vermilion border (upper lip) to a wide-open cleft extending into an incompletely formed nostril. It may be present on either one or both sides of the upper lip. Associated frequently with a cleft lip is a cleft of the palate. The occurrence of this abnormality is about one in 800 births.

The plastic surgeon is usually notified soon after a birth by the obstetrician or pediatrician. Evaluation is performed to determine the presence of other abnormalities, the general condition of the patient, and special feeding problems that may arise because the cleft lip/palate patient is usually unable to nurse properly. Next, a candid discussion with the parents is in order. Are they acquainted with this deformity? They are reassured (not falsely) that the appearance can be greatly improved. After the parents have recovered somewhat from the initial shock and the cleft lip patient is able to feed, the infant is discharged from the hospital to the home under a pediatrician's care. Usually at about six weeks of age, if the patient is healthy and is gaining weight consistently, photographs are then taken and the cleft lip is reconstructed.

Bernie was usually up at 6:30 am and at the hospital before 8:00 am to make the rounds, to visit previously operated on patients. He would then check any patients scheduled for morning surgery and consult with both the pediatrician and anesthesiologist. A cleft lip surgical procedure, under general anesthesia, usually takes about an hour, depending upon the complexity of the problem. When surgery was completed, the patient would be transferred to the recovery room for postoperative care. Bernie would then prepare for the next surgical procedure of the morning. After that surgical procedure had been completed, a third could be scheduled if there was time. After finishing the schedule for the morning, he would again make the rounds, checking on all of his postoperative patients. This effectively ended the day at the hospital, barring any emergencies.

By this time, he would be ready for lunch either at the hospital or at a restaurant near his office. Sometimes the schedule was such that there was no time for lunch. He would then leave the hospital and usually arrive at his office by about 1 pm where his secretary briefed him on the office schedule and any calls from doctors, patients or others. He then reviewed the mail and would begin to see patients at about two o'clock. Recently operated on patients are seen for in-office procedures such as dressing of their wounds and suture removal. He would follow other patients postoperatively for weeks and sometimes for months. The cleft lip patient would be seen at about the fifth day for removal of skin sutures. Because he could not eat normally, the patient would be fed with a special dropper and the wound kept clean. After all the sutures had been removed, the patient was allowed to nurse from a bottle. As soon as possible, the patient was put on a normal diet for his or her age. During the immediate postoperative period, splints were kept on the arms so that the patient would not be able to touch the wound. The patient was followed up periodically for any necessary "touch up" surgical procedures. There would be continued discussions with the parents.

New patients would also be seen during office hours for various problems. Thus, some surgeries under local anesthesia on an out-patient basis were done at the office for the removal of, for example, small tumors of the skin. Bernie, like all physicians, had to be prepared for emergencies at all hours of the day and night.

(B) Aesthetic Surgery: Face/Neck Lift

This aesthetic procedure is performed on female and on some male patients with redundant face and neck tissues. Briefly, loose skin of the face and neck is dissected free from the underlying tissue and advanced upward and backward. The excess tissue is excised and the wound sutured.

The patient would be first seen in the office to determine the patient's desires and to make an evaluation of the patient's needs as well as his or her psychological makeup and health. If the patient plans to lose weight this should be done before the contemplated surgery. Cigarette smoking and anticoagulants are to be discontinued for a definite period before surgery. Photographs are taken. The family physician must give approval of the patient's physical condition for surgery. The advantages and disadvantages of the procedure are discussed in detail so that the patient will not have any false hopes. The patient is also given medication to be taken the night before surgery and again the next morning to allay apprehension.

Bernie would arrive at about 7.30 am for an 8.00 am surgery. Discussions would then be taken up with an anesthesiologist for standby anesthesia. Bernie would use local anesthesia and the anesthesiologist would provide a supplement of light general anesthesia. The patient would usually be semiconscious and able to respond when necessary. Bernie would then prepare the surgical area by removing a minimal amount of hair and marking lines for the incision. Typically, a blood transfusion would not be needed. Since this was usually a three to three and a half-hour long procedure, Bernie would not schedule another such lengthy operation for the same day. The wound would be dressed, the patient's condition evaluated, and the patient transferred to the recovery room. After a day or so, the patient could be discharged to home or to a nursing facility. The wound would be dressed and the sutures subsequently removed. Usually after about 10 days, the patient would able to resume daily activities.

Many of the present-day surgical procedures, some common, others more uncommon, were not available to Bernie at the time of his practice. He ended his long surgical career before such specialties as liposuction, microvascular surgery, body sculpturing, botox and a host of other procedures had been fully developed.

Chapter 31

A DAY IN THE LIFE OF A BIOLOGICAL SCIENTIST

O ver a span of more than 60 years, Bernie's research interests have been primarily in bones and teeth that can be viewed as permanent recorders of both health and disease. Bones are about 65% and teeth about 98% calcified. Because of the different mechanisms of calcification, teeth are essentially immutable. That is, they are quite resistant to injury and environmental insult, although not totally. A wide variety of experimentation was performed on both bone and teeth for different purposes, different experiences and different results. This has led to more than 200 publications in refereed journals and books. Much of this work has received local, national and international recognition. A select group of experiments will be reviewed here, each illustrating a specific technique and providing particular information. After three years of broad clinical experience in general plastic and reconstructive surgery with doctors Blair and Byars in St. Louis, subsequent basic research was directed toward the relationship of biological aspects with clinical practice. During this period and the following decades, the specialty of craniofacial biology and subsequently that of craniofacial surgery evolved.

The Four Stages in Bernard Sarnat's Research Career

1. Introduction

During the summer of 1931, Bernie worked with two full-time graduate students in physiology at the University of Chicago working for their Ph.D.'s. The study dealt with the effect of secretin on blood flow in the pancreas of the dog. These were intense experiments that lasted over eight to ten hour periods. This was Bernie's introduction into basic research and experimental methodology.

2. Development

This covered the period between 1937 and 1940 as a graduate student with Isaac Schour as his mentor. Bernie became deeply involved in experimental and clinical research devoted to both bones and teeth. In addition to his work at the University of Illinois Graduate School, he also cooperated with researchers at the University of Chicago School of Medicine and Rush Medical College. This resulted in a number of publications.[1-3] One of them[3] was accorded the prestigious Joseph A. Capp's award offered by the Institute of Medicine of Chicago.

3. Mentor

In 1946, Bernie returned to the University of Illinois College of Dentistry and as head of the then Department of Oral and Plastic Surgery, instituted a graduate program. All the graduate students were involved with basic research problems, which eventually resulted in publications primarily in basic science journals as well as receiving a Master of Science degree. A number of publications resulted[4-15] leading to national and international recognition. Research was also conducted with some of his colleagues. Much of this work contributed to the early development of the specialty of craniofacial biology.[16-20]

4. Mentor again

By 1956, Bernie left the University of Illinois and moved to Los Angeles where he has remained to the present time. He again initiated research at the Cedars of Lebanon Hospital Research Institute, at Mount Sinai Hospital Medical Center, at UCLA Dental Research Institute and Medical School. Once again he served as a mentor to graduate and college students as well as some of his colleagues. This led to further publications.[21–34]

Research Experiments

A wide variety of experiments were undertaken. In each instance a question was proposed and an answer sought. The design was initially conceived to generally elicit a yes or no answer, although this proved not to be the case in many instances. As often arises with the conduct of research, answers were not always forthcoming. Sometimes one would have to be satisfied with a "maybe" answer. Frequently, with the completion of an experiment, there would be unanswered questions. This would often lead to further research. No research day was ever the same. Each was different with different problems going in different directions. In some instances associations could be made between the basic science and clinical practice. In other instances there was no immediate clinical application; research was done to increase basic biological knowledge. Along the way with the basic findings of each project, there were invariably interesting and fascinating developments.

Only a few selected experiments will be discussed here, usually with some unexpected highlights. The following experiments will be considered in brief: (1) hibernation of ground squirrels; (2) the mandibular growth pattern in pigs; (3) the removal of the mandibular condyle in the rhesus monkey (*Macaca mulatta*); (4) growth of the nasal bone and nasal septum in rabbits; and (5) growth of the turtle shell.

1. Hibernation

This was undertaken in conjunction with a member of the Department of Medicine at the University of Chicago. The purpose of the experiment was to quantitatively determine the extent of hibernation of the ground squirrel (*Citellus tridecemlineatus*). The animals were obtained from students on the University of Wisconsin, Madison campus. The state paid a bounty of $0.25 per animal and the researchers paid an additional $0.25 so that the students received $0.50 per animal that they sent in. The animals were of unknown age. They were given an intraperitoneal injection of a vital stain (alizarin red S), which was deposited in most calcifying structures such as dentin and bone. The animals were deprived of food and water for 48 hours and then placed in individual cages in a large walk-in refrigerator at 2°C to 5°C. This experiment took place during the hot summer months in Chicago and the investigators while working in the refrigerator from 30 to 45 minutes or so, had their overcoats, hats, ear muffs, scarves and gloves on. They entered the refrigerator every two to three days to check on the animals. If they were in hibernation they would be in the fetal position. They could unfurl them and the animal would return to the fetal position. They soon learned that the warmth of their hands would tend to awaken the animals, so henceforth gloves were worn. At the end of some of the experiments, which lasted as long as 59 days, after the animals were removed from the refrigerator and came out of hibernation, a second injection of alizarin red S was given. Some of the animals hibernated for 100% of the time and the rate of dentin formation was as low as 12% compared to the 100% of the controls. The ground squirrel incisor is a continuously growing, erupting and calcifying structure.

In some instances the animal would awaken, look around and urinate red from the alizarin red S on the paper lining the cage. In some other instances, an animal would inadvertently place its leg through the cage into another nearby cage and it was found that the leg had been eaten by the other animal totally bare down of the bone. This, of course, was an example of bloodless refrigeration anesthesia. This experiment on hibernation was first reported in 1941 probably well before NASA's involvement with the space program, raising the question of whether man can also be induced to hibernate. However, as caveat, it should be added that there are only very few animals that truly hibernate.

2. Mandibular growth

In addition to the use of vital stains for the study of growth of bones and dentin (as mentioned in the section on hibernation above), another important method is the use of radio-opaque 2–3 mm dental amalgam (the same filling material used for human teeth) as implants in growing bone(s). A 2 to 3 mm hole was drilled in bone and the radio opaque dental amalgam inserted. This procedure can be used in two different ways. One method is to insert two or more implants within a single bone as was done in the mandible,[35] the nasal bone[36] and the turtle plastron shell.[34] These implants maintained their same relationship to each other during the entire period of growth. Superimposed tracings of serial radiographs demonstrate the growth pattern of a single bone. A second procedure was to study sutural bone growth with amalgam implants placed on either side of a suture. Serial X-ray studies determine the growth pattern. This was demonstrated in five facial sutures in *Macaca mulatta*,[37] the frontonasal suture in rabbits[38] and the turtle shell.[34]

A study was undertaken at the University of Illinois in Chicago of the growth of the mandible in the pig.[35] One of the earliest works by Hunter published in 1778 was a comparison of human mandibles of different ages. Our modern study using serial radiography was a much more sophisticated and accurate one. Since this experiment was conducted in Chicago, Bernie and his graduate student were able to obtain nine weanling Hampshire pigs from a local stockyard. They weighed on average 20 pounds each. A special head holder was designed so that each time an X-ray picture was taken the animal's head could be positioned accurately. The animals were under the care of the animal hospital at the University of Illinois in Chicago and the Department of Agriculture. Serial X-ray pictures were taken periodically. The pigs grew rapidly and soon had to be moved out of the animal hospital because of their size to a nearby building for care. This building turned out to be a deserted synagogue, a fine place for two Jewish researchers who could not read the Hebrew descriptions on the outside of the building. The animals grew rapidly and by 12 weeks they weighed an average of 109 pounds each. They became difficult to handle and had essentially outgrown the head holder. So it was proposed to terminate the experiment of these healthy normal pigs. It was suggested that roast pig be served at a faculty dinner to demonstrate one of the unexpected byproducts of research.

The findings in this experiment demonstrated some important basic facts about the growth pattern of the mandible. From a clinical point of view it illustrated some of the do's and don'ts for surgery of the mandible (this will be made clearer in the next section).

3. Surgical removal of the mandibular condyle

The findings of the growth pattern of the mandible showed that the site of the upper aspect of the mandible (the condylar head), the part that articulates with the temporal bone of the skull (the glenoid fossa), was an important site of growth. So the question arose as to what would happen if the condyles were removed. This was done in young monkeys (*Macaca mulatta*). The final postoperative findings were quite severe. There was an extreme facial asymmetry, the mandible was less developed on the operated-on side, the mid-face which had not been surgically involved demonstrated a lack of growth and asymmetry, and the temporal bone was not as large as on the unoperated-on side. In addition, there was less lateral growth of the mandible.[39,40] This experiment was later carried out in adult squirrel monkeys with similar results.[41]

This research was awarded second prize in 1950 by the Plastic Surgical Educational Foundation in an international competition.

First prize was won by a Chinese national, third prize by an Argentinean and fourth prize by a British subject.

Housing of the monkeys presented something of a problem. Several of the monkeys had escaped their cages and managed to go through the open windows and were running up and down a ledge on the third floor of the building about one block long. Students and people outside were watching with amusement as the animal keepers tried to catch the monkeys. After a number of futile attempts they were re-captured. So now the monkeys, instead of being placed into cages with a simple lock, were put into cages with combination locks. After a while the monkeys figured out the combination lock and escaped again. They were then constrained in the cages using a padlock with a cover over the key slot. They solved this problem as well and were soon loose again. Finally the monkeys had to be collared and chained to their cages. But for a month, the investigators were getting tired and frustrated from the numerous calls indicating that: "your monkeys are loose and running along the 3rd floor ledge again".

4. Growth of the nasal bone and nasal septum

The experiments on the nasal bone and the nasal septum in the rabbit contributed significant clinical knowledge to rhinoplasty or cosmetic operations on the nose. Two studies were involved. The first one was concerned with the growth pattern of the nasal bone. It was probably the first report depicting this growth pattern.[42] This report received the 1980 Cottle award offered by the American Rhinologic Society. In the second study it was demonstrated that if too much of the nasal septum was removed, a severe deformity of the nose and face could result. Clinically, these two experiments were important in that they showed that in nasal plastic surgery, fracture of the nasal bones did not affect the growth of the nose but removal of too much septum could end in a negative result.

There was an interesting incident in the laboratory. On Friday, December 23rd, sometime in the early 1960's, Bernie had decided to conclude the rabbit experiment on which septal surgery had been performed. He injected the otherwise normal rabbits with intracardiac Nembutal to euthanize the rabbits. His interests lay only in the heads and not the rest of the body. The laboratory workers requested the bodies as they were having a Christmas Eve party that Saturday. Bernie, of course, agreed. That Christmas Eve party was a huge success — with much vodka and plenty of rabbit. When Bernie returned to the lab to check on his remaining animals on Monday morning he found that half of the laboratory personnel were absent and the remaining personnel were sluggishly dragging their bodies around. The combination of Nembutal and alcohol had evidently had a profound synergistic effect.

5. Growth of the turtle shell

For several years Bernie presented a twelve-week graduate course on bone biology at UCLA, of two-hour duration weekly. During the course a discussion of the growth of turtle shell arose. This was of interest because the turtle is the only animal that has sutural growth not limited to the skull. Further, it is of interest that the turtle is unique in that it has the hard tissue on the outside and soft tissue on the inside in contrast to other living examples of *chordata* (animals with spinal chords). Thus, growth of the turtle shell could be compared with growth of the cranium. An experiment was set up that was similar to the study of the frontonasal suture[43] and the nasal bone.[44] Two radiopaque implants were inserted in four different bones. Thus, both sutural growth[34] and growth of an individual bone could be determined. Finally, a recent study also established that asymmetry was present in the growth of the turtle carapace.[45]

A graduate student had a two-year period to devote to this experiment. The initial thought was to obtain 50 turtles from a pet store. However, at just about that time, the State Department of Public Health negated the sale of pet turtles because of an outbreak of Salmonella infections. Therefore, disease-free turtles had to be located. After several months, a source of hatchling turtles was obtained from Northern California. The turtles were housed in eleven aquaria. It was soon discovered that the turtles had individual personalities. Some were more aggressive than others. This was particularly noted at feeding time. As a result, the turtles were then separated according to their aggressiveness. When the time for feeding occurred, the turtles seem to be fully aware and eager for the food. Initially, the inserted radiopaque implants did not remain in place so the implantation had to be delayed for several weeks until they were 58 days old when adequate ossification had occurred. At the end of two years the graduate student left and an undergraduate student was recruited. After 810 days the experiment was finally ended,

In this experiment, growth of the soft tissue influenced growth of the bony turtle shell. This was compared with growth of the brain and the cranium. Experiments have shown that the brain growth is the predominant force in determining the growth of the cranial bones in humans. This process is similar in the turtle and was a primary reason for its choice as an experimental model.

At the end of the twelve-week course mentioned earlier, there was a take-home open book question as part of the final examination. The question was as follows: Earth man and earth woman decide to live on the moon. A child is conceived and born on the moon. Describe the bony and musculature development of this child and contrast it with an earth-born child.

Chapter 32

A CAREER AS PLASTIC SURGEON AND RESEARCHER

Bernard G. Sarnat S.B., M.D., M.S., D.D.S., F.A.C.S., was born in 1912 in Chicago, a child of immigrant parents from Eastern Europe where his two older siblings were born. He was raised early on the Northwest side of Chicago, a predominantly Jewish neighborhood and subsequently on the Southside a predominantly Protestant/Catholic area.

Formative Years

There was no history of either surgeons or scientists in Bernie's family. At the young age of nine years Bernie had been influenced by his 19 year-old dental student brother to become an oral and plastic surgeon. This was 1921. Growing up he was interested in biology and science. He was an honor student in grammar school and high school and was awarded early admission to the undergraduate college of the University of Chicago with advanced college credit for certain high school courses.

At the University of Chicago he was exposed to basic science research. At the end of his junior year he took an undergraduate honors research course in physiology and did exceptionally well and thought of specializing in that area and getting a Ph.D. in Physiology. Nevertheless, his goal remained to subsequently obtain a dental degree and specialize in oral plastic surgery. At the medical school the faculty was composed of clinicians, many of whom were engaged in basic science research. This concept, of being both a clinician and a researcher, was readily embraced by Bernie.

Thus, he continued to pursue his studies toward medicine. His grades were probably somewhat above average in college but adequate enough to be admitted to the University of Chicago School of Medicine. At that time a student had two choices for the third and fourth clinical years: (1) to pursue studies at the well-established and famous clinically-oriented Rush Medical College on the Westside of Chicago with classes of more than a 100 students; or (2) consider the relatively new medical school on the university campus on the Southside, consisting of a research-oriented full-time clinical faculty. The class was limited to about 35 students. The latter institution appealed more to Bernie and he was fortunate in being one of those selected. Throughout his six but not the seventh year as a University of Chicago student, it was necessary to work in his father's drugstore just off the University of Chicago campus 30 hours a week, this being the years of the Great Depression of the 1930's. He asked to be relieved from work in the drugstore during his last year in medical school to be able to devote full-time to his studies. He never again worked in the drugstore.

During his undergraduate years, because of pressure from his older sister, he joined a social fraternity. As a result he became somewhat active on campus and became an all University intramural wrestling champion for two years. Because this increased the strain on his limited time schedule, he dropped out of the fraternity during his third year of college to devote more essential time to study.

After a wonderful year in an internship at the Los Angeles County General Hospital he stayed long enough to take and pass the California Medical State Board examination.

Later when he interviewed the deans of several dental schools he was planning to attend, Bernie had a triple program in mind. Yes, he wanted to obtain a doctor of dental surgery degree to further his goals of becoming an oral and plastic surgeon. But at the same time he wanted the opportunity to embark on a research career and also be engaged in teaching.

He then returned to Chicago and enrolled in the University of Illinois College of Dentistry and Graduate School, to conduct research under Dr. Isaac Schour. Bernie was positively attracted to Dr. Schour and an appropriate appointment was immediately arranged as a junior faculty member.

He was most fortunate in finding the ideal place to satisfy his goals at the University of Illinois College of Dentistry and Graduate School. Dr. Isaac Schour, who had bachelor's and Ph.D. degrees from the University of Chicago as well as a Doctor of Dental Surgery degree from the University of Illinois, was a foremost pioneer and world-famous researcher in dental histo-physiology and histo-pathology.

After three years of highly intensive work Bernie was awarded M.S. and D.D.S. degrees in 1940. In particular the three years with Dr. Schour were very important formative years for Bernie and provided the basis for significant research programs for the next 60 or more years. This is where and under whom Bernie began his initial basic research and clinical studies. Bernie was launched on what proved to be his entire future highly productive career. A close personal bond developed between Schour and Sarnat.

Significant research in his third year on the relationship of teeth to systemic disease resulted in Bernie receiving the highly coveted Joseph Capps prize offered by the Institute of Medicine of Chicago. This and other research papers proved to be among the early pioneering efforts in the development of the new specialty of craniofacial biology and subsequently its relationship to the developing specialty of craniofacial surgery. These efforts were further crystallized in the mid 1940's up to the present time.

Clinical and Biological Research

In pursuing his goal of becoming a plastic surgeon he devoted one year as a resident at Cook County Hospital in oral and plastic surgery and a subsequent year in general surgery at University

Hospital also in Chicago. This was followed by three very busy years learning the art and science of general plastic and reconstructive surgery in St. Louis as an assistant to the internationally-famous doctors Vilray P. Blair and Louis T. Byars. Bernie's clinical appointments were not only in the private practice office but also in the Department of Surgery at Washington University School of Medicine and Barnes Hospital. Subsequently, he was appointed full professor and head of the Department of Oral and Plastic surgery at St. Louis University School of Dentistry. After these further important developmental years Bernie returned to Chicago and established his private practice of plastic and reconstructive surgery. At this time he also became professor and head of the Department of Oral and Plastic Surgery in the College of Dentistry and also a professor in Plastic Surgery in the Medical School and also the Graduate School.

He now had the opportunity to further pursue his basic research program and this also included graduate students. In the ensuing 10 years, significant research was carried out in the general field of bone and craniofacial biology. With this research the Department of Oral and Plastic Surgery established both a national and international reputation. By 1955, Bernie found that as head of the department he was devoting more and more time to administration and less and less to research. Because of this and other factors he resigned from all his appointments, closed his office of the private practice of plastic and reconstructive surgery and moved the family to Los Angeles in December of 1955 to start life anew.

As a plastic surgeon with a basic science background, Bernie saw in his practice patients with a variety of both soft and hard tissue deformities which frequently were distributed over many parts of the body. Invariably there were many unanswered questions. In an attempt to find answers to these questions, Bernie returned to the laboratory and over the years conceived, designed, initiated, and carried out a series of experiments in regard to bone, teeth, cartilage and cartilage implants, in both young and adult animals (turtles, rats, gophers, lagomorphs, pigs, dogs, monkeys, and humans), for which he eventually received international recognition (Fig. 46,

Fig. 50 and Fig. 51). Each procedure had its advantages and disadvantages. Although an attempt was made to limit the number of variables and to obtain a definite yes or no answer, this was not always possible. His early research interests were in skeletal problems of a systemic nature. Later, one of the concerns was the effects of trauma, accidental or intentional (surgical), on the growth of bones. This was carried out by experimental surgical procedures. Eventually he directed his efforts principally toward local surgical experimentation as related to both normal and abnormal gross postnatal craniofacial and dental growth. Because of the wide variety of different structures, their interrelated individualities and the challenges presented by both the diversity of the sites of growth and the complexity of the skull and particularly the face, this will continue to be a challenging endeavor for researchers in the future.

Some Closing Thoughts

The last few years have been primarily devoted to the completion of two books. The first one is this biography. The second one is entitled: *Some Essays on Craniofacial Biology and Craniofacial Surgery*. This book was developed with James Bradley, M.D. as co-author and is now in press (Fig. 54).

Bernie always considered himself as a shy, somewhat self-effacing, quiet and modest person, happiest when he was in his professional office or laboratory. He was never a political person and as such never sought office; those he held were by invitation only. He served in various capacities, at one time or another, as Vice President of the University of Chicago School of Medicine Alumni Association; President of the University of Chicago Alumni Association of Greater Los Angeles; Program Chair of California Society of Plastic Surgeons; President of the Craniofacial Biology Group; President of the Beverly Hills Academy of Medicine; Secretary of the Research Committee and member of the Executive Committee Mt. Sinai Hospital, Los Angeles; Chief of Plastic Surgery, Cedars-Sinai Medical Center for more than 20 years; founding member and Chairman of the Plastic Surgery Research

Council; etc. Bernie also turned down offers such as President of the California Society of Plastic Surgeons, The Aesthetic Society and Vice-chair of the Cedars-Sinai Medical Staff. Bernie also restricted the number of professional organizations that he joined or was invited to join, and only considered those that he felt he might attend from time to time. He was simply not a joiner by temperament.

It is perhaps fitting to end this chapter with a citation from Harvey Zarem, M.D. former chief of plastic surgery at UCLA who said in 1987: "Dr. Sarnat is a proud but quietly humble man .... this award will call attention to his contributions in basic research, his care of children with deformities and his especially unique role in the teaching and training of dental as well as medical students. And may I add, to the teaching of all of us in plastic surgery."

CHAPTER NOTES

Introduction

1. Lestrel, Pete E., Sarnat, B. G. and McNabb, E. G. Fourier analysis of carapace shape: Growth of the Turtle *Chrysemys scripta*. *J. Dent. Res.* **66**:347 (1987).
2. Lestrel, P. E., Sarnat, B. G. and McNabb, E. G. Carapace growth of the Turtle Chrysemys scripta: A longitudinal study of shape using Fourier Analysis. *Anat. Anz.* (Jena) **168**:135–143 (1989).
3. Lestrel, P. E., Sarnat, B. G., Read, D. W., Wolfe, C. A and Bodt, A. Three-dimensional characterization of eye orbit shape: Fourier Descriptors. *Am. J. Phys. Anthrop. Suppl.* **16**:134 (1993).
4. Lestrel, P. E., Wolfe, C. A., Read, D. W. and Sarnat, B. G. A numerical analysis of the rabbit orbital margin: Three-dimensional Fourier-Descriptors. *J. Dent. Res.* **74**:580 (1995).
5. Lestrel, P. E., Read, D. W. and Wolfe, C. A. Size and shape of the rabbit eye orbit: 3-D Fourier Descriptors. In: P. E. Lestrel (ed.). *Fourier Descriptors and Their Applications in Biology.* Cambridge University Press, New York (1997).

Chapter 1. Background

1. Twain, M. Concerning the Jews. *Harper's Magazine*, **99**:727–535 (1899).
2. The term "anti-Semitism" did not exist until the work of Wilhelm Marr, a German agitator, who coined it in 1879 (Davidowicz, 1975). However, "anti-Jewishness" is the preferred term here because the word "Semite" refers to both Jews and other cultural groups.

3. Davidowicz, L. S. *The War Against the Jews — 1933–1945*. Holt, Rinehart and Winston, New York (1975).
4. This was a number often quite out of proportion to their non-Jewish (gentile) counterparts, when population figures are examined. Additionally, this was not just limited to the fields of science and medicine, but also extended to the arts and letters including entertainment fields such as the movies and the stage (Gilbert, 2001).
5. Gilbert, M. *The Jews in the Twentieth Century*. Schocken Books, New York (2001).
6. www.jewishsf.com Retrieved October 4, 2002.
7. From the start of the Nobel Prize until 1933, Germany won more Nobel prizes than any other country, about 30% of the total. Of Germany's share, Jews were responsible for nearly a third and in medicine fully one half (Johnson, 1987).
8. Johnson, P. *A History of the Jews*. Harper and Row Publishers, New York (1987).
9. Dobbs, S. M. As the Nobel Prize marks centennial, Jews constitute 1/5 of laureates. Retrieved December 13, 2001: http://www.jewishsf.com/bk011012/sfp18.shtml.
10. Medawar, J. and Pyke, D. *Hitler's gift*. Arcade Publishing, New York (2000).
11. It should be noted that although the persecution of Jews in Germany was common at times throughout the millennium of Jewish settlement there, conditions had improved from the 1860's to the 1920's (Cutler, 1996). Jews were also favorably received in the United Kingdom, where they flourished. They were elected to parliament in 1858, entered university in 1871 and achieved full emancipation in 1890 (Con-Sherbok, 1994).
12. Cutler, I. *The Jews of Chicago: From Shtetl to Suburb*. University of Illinois Press, Chicago (1996).
13. Cohn-Sherbok, D. *Atlas of Jewish History*. Routledge, London (1994).

Chapter 2. Tsarist Russia

1. Eban, A. *Heritage: Civilization of the Jews*. Summit Books, New York (1984).

2. Ben-Sasson, H. H. (ed.). *A History of the Jewish People*. Harvard University Press, Cambridge (1976).

3. Ettinger, S. The modern period. In: Ben-Sasson, H. H. (ed.). *A History of the Jewish People*. Harvard University Press, Cambridge (1976).

4. Early in the 14th century, these were two separate entities: The Kingdom of Poland and the Grand Principality of Lithuania. These two initially merged into one Kingdom in 1386 for security against the Teutonic knights. Technically, they remained separate states until the Union of Lublin (1565), after which they re-merged to form the Kingdom of Poland. The Kingdom of Poland then expanded its borders eastward at the expense of Muscovite Russia to assume its largest extent in 1634–1635 (Hupchick and Cox (2001).

5. Sorkin, D. into the modern world. In: Lange de, N. (ed.). *The Illustrated History of the Jewish People*. Harcourt Brace and Company, New York (1997).

6. As Jews were distinctive from their Slav counterparts, in terms of dress, language and especially religion, they were viewed as other foreigners and treated accordingly; that is, with suspicion, hence the need for restrictions.

7. Note: At this time all Jews were effectively Orthodox. The ideas of the Enlightenment that later influenced Judaism and produced the largely secular Jew, were not present until much later.

8. Cutler, I. *The Jews of Chicago: From Shtetl to Suburb*. University of Illinois Press, Chicago (1996).

9. Grey, I. *Catherine the Great* (Autocrat and Empress of all Russia). Hodder and Stoughton, London (1961).

10. Hupchick, D. P. and Cox, H. E. *The Palgrave Concise Historical Atlas of Eastern Europe*. Palgrave, New York (2001).

11. Cross, A. G. Russia looks west. In: Constable, G. (ed.). *Winds of Revolution*. (Time Frame AD 1700–1800). Time-Life Books, Alexandria, Virginia (1990).

12. Stanislaw II reluctantly accepted the Polish kingship believing that it would lead to marriage with Catherine II. He was to be sorely disappointed as Catherine II had other plans. After the 1795 Third Partition, he was forced to retire and took up the study of botany. He died in St. Petersburg in 1797 (Cross, 1990; Grey, 1961).

13. Barnavi, E. (ed.). *A Historical Atlas of the Jewish People*. Schocken Books, New York (1992).

14. Channon, J. *The Penguin Historical Atlas of Russia*. Penguin Books, London (1996).

15. Eliach, Y. *There Once was a World* (A 900-year Chronicle of the *Shtetl* of Eishyshok). Little Brown and Company, New York (1998).

16. Sachar, A. L. *A History of the Jews*, 4th ed. Alfred A. Knopf, Publisher, New York (1953).

17. Although Warsaw, the Polish capital, fell to Russian troops in 1795, it was allotted to the Prussians via treaty.

18. While Jews had settled in the Kingdom of Poland and the Grand Duchy in Lithuania since the 14th century, they had been largely barred from Muscovite Russia for about 300 years, from the latter part of the 15th century until the end of the 18th century (Ettinger, 1976).

19. The nobility in Russia, as in Poland, had arrogated power to themselves always at the expense of the serfs.

20. She was fully aware that the conditions that led the French peasants to revolt were also present in Russia.

Chapter 3. The Pale of Settlement

1. The commonly used euphemism of a 'Jewish problem' had its roots in the historical hostility of the Russian Orthodox Church toward Jews, their distinctive dress, customs and language (Yiddish) exhibited by Eastern European Jews, which identified them as 'foreigners', foreigners who could never become Russians.

2. Lipman, D. Gates to Jewish Heritage: The Creation of the Pale of Settlement. Retrieved September 12, 2001: http://www.jewish-gates.org/history/jewhis/three.stm (2000).

3. Ettinger, S. The modern period. In: Ben-Sasson, H. H. (ed.). *A History of the Jewish People*. Harvard University Press, Cambridge (1976).

4. Sachar, A. L. *A History of the Jews*, 4th ed. Alfred A. Knopf, Publisher, New York (1953).

5. Grayzel, S. *A History of the Jews*. The Jewish Publication Society of America, Philadelphia (1947).

6. Kouchel, B. I. Tracing Jewish Ancestors. Retrieved November 21, 2001: http://www.jewishgen.org/infofiles/ru-pale.txt (1990).

7. Eliach, Y. *There Once was a World* (A 900-year Chronicle of the *Shtetl* of Eishyshok). Little Brown and Company, New York (1998).
8. Pale is derived from the Latin *palus* meaning 'stake'. It is an archaic English word for an enclosure limited by a border or boundary (Webster, 1972).
9. In 1516, Jews were not permitted to leave the Venice Jewish quarter at night, leading to the creation of the first ghetto (Eban, 1984).
10. The 1804 decree promised the right to settle anywhere in the country, the granting of agricultural land and permission to manufacture alcohol, if they converted to Christianity, few did (Ettinger, 1976).
11. Johnson, P. *A History of the Jews.* Harper and Row Publishers, New York (1987).

Chapter 4. The Napoleonic Wars

1. Hupchick, D. P. and Cox, H. E. *The Palgrave Concise Historical Atlas of Eastern Europe.* Palgrave, New York (2001).
2. The agreement was to allow Alexander I of Russia a free hand to expand westward and add Sweden to its Baltic possessions. However, Russian fortunes in regard to Sweden came to nothing with Napoleon's attack on Russia in 1812 (Carter, 1997). Napoleon attacked Russia without first declaring war, a pattern that was to be repeated by Hitler in 1941.
3. Carter, R. The last Tsars. In: Benn, A. (ed.). *Russia* (Insight Guides). Houghton Mifflin Company, Boston (1997).
4. The name 'Poland' was not used at the insistence of Tsar Alexander I (Hupchick and Cox, 2001).
5. Seltzer, R. M. *Jewish People, Jewish Thought: The Jewish Experience in History.* Macmillan Publishing Co., Inc., New York (1980).
6. Lange de, N. *Atlas of the Jewish World.* Facts on File, Inc., New York (1984).
7. Sachar, A. L. *A History of the Jews,* 4th ed. Alfred A. Knopf, Publisher, New York (1953).
8. Ettinger, S. The modern period. In: Ben-Sasson, H. H. (ed.). *A History of the Jewish People.* Harvard University Press, Cambridge (1976).
9. Cohn-Sherbok, D. *Atlas of Jewish History.* Routledge, London (1994).

10. Gartner, L. *History of the Jews in Modern Times*. Oxford University Press, Oxford (2001).

11. Kniesmeyer, J. and Brecher, D. C. Beyond the Pale: A Life in the Pale of Settlement. Retrieved September 12, 2001: http://www.friends-partners.org/partners/beyond-the-pale/english/30/html (1995a).

12. Leeson, D. Military Conscription in the 19th Century. Retrieved November 21, 2001. http://www.jewishgen.org/infofiles/rupale.txt (1995).

13. Refers to the so-called canton-schools run by the military.

14. This included the violation of dietary restrictions such as the forced consumption of pork.

15. The policy remained on the books until 1917 when the Bolsheviks repealed it.

16. Grayzel, S. *A History of the Jews*. The Jewish Publication Society of America, Philadelphia (1947).

17. Gilbert, M. *The Jews in the Twentieth Century*. Schocken Books, New York (2001).

18. Prevailing social conditions of the peasants or serfs prior to Alexander II were virtually slavery. Serfs were owned by landlords and treated as animals or property. After emancipation in 1861, things initially appeared to improve but that turned out to be illusionary. In fact, conditions worsened largely until the collapse of the Tsarist regime in 1917.

19. Parker, G. *The World an Illustrated History*. Harper and Row Publishers, New York (1986).

20. Castelló, E. R. and Kapon, U. M. *The Jews and Europe*. Henry Holt and Company, New Jersey (1994).

21. Barnavi, E. (ed.). *A Historical Atlas of the Jewish People*. Schocken Books, New York (1992).

22. One factor that also contributed to increased anti-Jewishness was the increasing perception of being citizens of nation states. This rise in nationalism acted to heighten tensions between the dominant populations and the minority groups, Jews among them.

23. As Gartner (2001) indicated, the decline of liberal European political ideas in the West was replaced with the rise of nationalism, aggressive imperialism, socialism, the union movement, Social Darwinism, as well as anti-Jewishness.

Chapter 5. Initiation of Pogroms

1. There were two other anti-Jewish incidents, one in 1821 and the other in 1859, but these had little in common with those pogroms that occurred in the 1880's (Lambroza, 1987).
2. Lambroza, S. Jewish responses to pogroms in late Imperial Russia. In: Reinharz, J. (ed.). *Living with Antisemitism,* University Press of New England, Hanover (1987).
3. Alexander II was assassinated by members of a revolutionary terrorist organization called Narodnya Volya (The People's Will).
4. Grayzel, S. *A History of the Jews.* The Jewish Publication Society of America, Philadelphia (1947).
5. Johnson, P. *A History of the Jews.* Harper and Row Publishers, New York (1987).
6. Sachar, A. L. *A History of the Jews,* 4th ed. Alfred A. Knopf, Publisher, New York (1953).
7. According to Sachar (1953), Pobedonostsev despised parliamentary institutions and his fanaticism as head of the Orthodox Church earned him the title of the "second Torquemada".
8. The evidence in regard to the actual number of pogroms is conflicting (Gartner, 2001).
9. It has long been accepted that the Russian government was, in part, responsible for the pogroms. However, that view has recently been altered. The regime was actually surprised by the pogroms and viewed revolutionary agitators as responsible. Nevertheless, some local officials tolerated and clearly encouraged the outbreaks of violence (Gartner, 2001).
10. Gartner, L. *History of the Jews in Modern Times.* Oxford University Press, Oxford (2001).
11. A particularly severe 1882 pogrom occurred in the town of Balta on the Russian-Rumanian border (Ettinger, 1976).
12. Ettinger, S. The modern period. In: Ben-Sasson, H. H. (ed.). *A History of the Jewish People.* Harvard University Press, Cambridge (1976).
13. In 1882, Ignatiev was replaced by Dmitri Tolstoy, who declared that pogroms would not be tolerated. The number of pogroms sharply decreased for a number of years (Ettinger, 1976; Gartner, 2001).
14. The laws prohibited Jews from settling in villages (even in the Pale), opening shops on Sundays, etc. These regulations as official policy

were then used as justification by local bureaucrats to harass Jews (Ettinger, 1976). These May Laws actually remained on the books until the end of the Tsarist regime in 1917 (Gartner, 2001).

15. Kniesmeyer, J. and Brecher, D. C. Beyond the Pale: A Life in the Pale of Settlement. Retrieved September 12, 2001: http://www.friends-partners.org/partners/beyond-the-pale/english/30/html (1995a).

16. Kniesmeyer, J. and Brecher, D. C. Beyond the Pale: Renewed Oppression — the "May Laws". Retrieved September 12, 2001: http://www.friends-partners.org/partners/beyond-the-pale/english/34/html (1995b).

17. Cutler, I. *The Jews of Chicago: From Shtetl to Suburb*. University of Illinois Press, Chicago (1996).

Chapter 6. Jewish Migration

1. Sachar, A. L. *A History of the Jews*, 4th ed. Alfred A. Knopf, Publisher, New York (1953).

2. Cutler, I. *The Jews of Chicago: From Shtetl to Suburb*. University of Illinois Press, Chicago (1996).

3. Eliach, Y. *There Once was a World* (A 900-year Chronicle of the *Shtetl* of Eishyshok). Little Brown and Company, New York (1998).

4. Gartner, L. *History of the Jews in Modern Times*. Oxford University Press, Oxford (2001).

5. The Pale had a high birthrate of 40 per 1000 population, which more than offset emigration. Thus, of the two solutions suggested by the leadership of St. Petersburg, emigration or emancipation, neither of which improved the conditions of the Pale (Lambroza, 1987)

6. Lambroza, S. Jewish Responses to Pogroms in Late Imperial Russia. In: Reinharz, J. (ed.). *Living with Antisemitism*, University Press of New England, Hanover (1987).

7. Lange de, N. *Atlas of the Jewish World*. Facts on File, Inc., New York (1984).

8. Ettinger, S. The modern period. In: Ben-Sasson, H. H. (ed.). *A History of the Jewish People*. Harvard University Press, Cambridge (1976).

9. Johnson, P. *A History of the Jews*. Harper and Row Publishers, New York (1987).

10. Parker, G. *The World an Illustrated History.* Harper and Row Publishers, New York (1986).

11. Kishinev was also the location of where the Russian secret police (the Cheka, forerunner of the KBG) published the 1905 forgery entitled *Protocols of the Learned Elders of Zion,* an anti-Jewish propaganda tract supposedly providing guidelines for eventual Jewish world domination. The document was intended to demonstrate the Jewish threat to the Russian Empire under Tsar Nicholas II. Nicholas II not fooled, wrote on the document, 'A worthy cause is not defended by evil means' (Johnson, 1987).

12. Pogrom statistics seem to be quite variable. One source has more than 300 killed, thousands wounded, 1500 homes and shops plundered and 40,000 people left without property or means of work in Kishinev (Potok, 1996). Another source has 45 killed and 1,300 shops and homes plundered (Kniesmeyer and Brecher, 1995c).

13. Property damage in Kishinev was estimated at more than three million rubles (Lambroza, 1987).

14. It is estimated that the total destruction of property during 1903–1906 pogroms exceeded 57 million rubles in the Pale (Lambroza, 1987).

15. Renck, E. S. *Piesk and Most, a History of two Cities.* Retrieved November 20, 2001: http://www.jewishgen.org/Yizkor/Piaski/piesk.html (1975).

16. Population figures from 1897 show that Skidel, located about 37km from Piesk, had a Jewish population of 2222, while Piesk had a Jewish population of 1615. Both towns were comparable in terms of mercantile trades such as shoemaker, tailor, carpenter, etc. (Renck, 1975).

17. Cohn-Sherbok, D. *Atlas of Jewish History.* Routledge, London (1994).

Chapter 7. Bolshevik Revolution

1. Ironically, the Russian word *Bolsheviki* means the majority, which, initially, they decidedly were not (Cunliffe, 1974).

2. Cunliffe, M. *The Age of Expansion 1848–1917.* G. & C. Merriam Company, Publishers, Springfield, Massachusetts (1974).

3. The White Russians represented varied groups who wanted a return to the old economic order, and viewed the Bolsheviks as a threat. Moreover, they viewed Jews as largely pro-Bolshevik (Sachar, 1953).

4. Sachar, A. L. *A History of the Jews,* 4th ed. Alfred A. Knopf, Publisher, New York (1953).

5. During the ensuing Civil War in the Ukraine, an estimated 60,000–70,000 Jews were murdered (Johnson, 1987). Again, this number is quite variable, one source estimating the number to be 100,000, possibly as high as 250,000 (Sachar, 1953). Another source suggests a range from 31,000 to 150,000 (Gartner, 2001).

6. Gartner, L. *History of the Jews in Modern Times.* Oxford University Press, Oxford (2001).

7. Reference should be made to Marx and Engel's *Communist Manifesto* (1848) among numerous other works.

8. He was actually a Jewish intellectual by the name of Lev Bronstein (Cunliffe, 1974).

9. Johnson, P. *A History of the Jews.* Harper and Row Publishers, New York (1987).

10. Although Lenin's mother's father was a Jewish physician who converted to Christianity, this fact was kept secret (Gartner, 2001).

11. Ettinger, S. The modern period. In: Ben-Sasson, H. H. (ed.). *A History of the Jewish People.* Harvard University Press, Cambridge (1976).

12. Potok, C. *The Gates of November* (Chronicles of the Slepak Family). Alfred A. Knopf, Publisher, New York (1996).

13. The plight of Soviet Jewry since 1953 has now been widely publicized but is beyond the scope of this book. The following references are recommended for further reading: Sachar (1985) and Potok (1996).

14. Only from 1926 to 1935 with the regime of Joseph Pilsudski as the first president of Poland (who was not anti-Jewish), did conditions for Jews improve. Before and afterwards, conditions remained deplorable (Gartner, 2001).

15. Cassel, D. Poland: In Solidarity with Jews? Retrieved December 16, 2001: http://www.law.northwestern.edu/depts/clinic/ihr/hrcomments/1995/june21-95.html (1995).

Chapter 8. Emigration to the United States

1. Gartner, L. *History of the Jews in Modern Times.* Oxford University Press, Oxford (2001).
2. Lange de, N. *Atlas of the Jewish World.* Facts on File, Inc., New York (1984).
3. Ettinger, S. The modern period. In: Ben-Sasson, H. H. (ed.). *A History of the Jewish People.* Harvard University Press, Cambridge (1976).
4. Cutler, I. *The Jews of Chicago: From Shtetl to Suburb.* University of Illinois Press, Chicago (1996).
5. Sachar, H. M. *Diaspora.* Harper and Row Publishers, New York (1985).
6. DellaPergola, S. World Jewish Population, 2000. Retrieved December 16, 2001: http://sites.huji.ac.il/jcj/dmg_worldjpop.html.

Chapter 9. A New Century

1. Although the Wright brothers (1903) proved that human flight was feasible, the impact was largely negligible until the advent of the First World War.
2. The discovery of oil in Tulsa, Oklahoma (1910) eventually allowed the automobile to become the predominant form of public transportation.
3. The cost for steerage was as low as $12 for a voyage from Italy (Britten, L. and Mathless, 1998).
4. Britten, L. and Mathless, P (eds.). *Dawn of the Century (1900–1910).* Time-Life Books, Inc., Alexandria, Virginia (1998).
5. The Economist: Dec. 21st, 2000.
6. Time Magazine: April 13, 1998.
7. Retrieved September 21, 2006 http://www.albertsons.com
8. Constable, G. (ed.). Gateway to the New World. In: *America comes of Age.* (TimeFrame AD 1900–1925). Time-Life Books, Inc., Alexandria, Virginia (1989).
9. A rate of 22 cents an hour, working 12 hours a day for 6 days a week, results in a paycheck of $15.84 a week.
10. The Triangle Shirtwaist factory fire of 1911, one of the many sweatshops in the New York garment industry, claimed the lives of

146 young women, Eastern European immigrants. That disaster eventually led to better working conditions, factory safety and building codes.

Chapter 10. Roots in Belarus

1. Unfortunately, little is available in the historical archives regarding the maternal side of the family lineage.
2. The name Sarnatzky with the ending (-zky) was also spelled with the ending (-sky).
3. Hugle, L. Sarnatzky Descendants. Retrieved September 12, 2001 from the World Wide Web: http://www.shtetlinks.jewishgen.org/skidel/sarntzk.htm (1999a).
4. Hugle, L. Town without Memory. Retrieved September 12, 2001 from the World Wide Web: http://www.shtetlinks.jewishgen.org/skidel/96travel.htm (1999b).
5. It has been estimated that around 900 such villages existed.
6. Note that the name Gittle was also spelled Gitla. The presence of such various spellings is not unusual and can be found throughout the archive data.
7. Hugle, L. Skidel History. Retrieved September 12, 2001 from the World Wide Web: http://www.shtetlinks.jewishgen.org/skidel/history.htm (1999c).

Chapter 11. Emigration to Chicago

1. Hugle, L. Sarnatzky Descendants. Retrieved September 12, 2001 from the World Wide Web: http://www.shtetlinks.jewishgen.org/skidel/sarntzk.htm (1999a).
2. Isadore was born in 1878 but claimed it was 1880. Upon arrival in the United States, it was common practice for immigrants to give a younger age since this could lead to a cheaper insurance policy.
3. Such retail stores were common at the time. They sold besides sundries, knives, tobacco goods, etc.
4. Bernie was actually working 30 hours a week there, from 6.00 pm to 12.00 midnight on Fridays and from 12.00 noon to 12.00 midnight on Saturdays and Sundays, leaving precious little time for study.

5. Drugstores at that time contained a soda fountain, sold tobacco products, candy, wine, liquor, cosmetics, and other sundries as well as a pharmacy for filling prescriptions.

Chapter 13. Elementary Lessons

1. This pattern of name change, especially for those of Jewish ancestry, was not uncommon. The author's parents first immigrated from Nazi Germany to Ecuador in 1938 and subsequently to the United States in 1948. The author's family name was Lichtenstern, which was first changed to Estrella (the rendering of the German word for star into Spanish) and then further altered to Lestrel.
2. The armistice that ended World War One was not signed until November 11, 1918. The actual armistice was signed on the 11th day, at the 11th hour and the 11th minute.
3. Bernie does not recall their identity.

Chapter 14. Growing Up in Chicago

1. This family was considered by some, who felt superior as city dwellers, to be *Landsleit* or rural folk in contrast to townsfolk.
2. Calvin Coolidge, 30th President of the United States (1923–1929). Although Coolidge was known to be an effective public speaker, in private, he was a man of few words and was therefore commonly referred to as "Silent Cal."
3. The Blackstone Rangers were Chicago's most infamous gang. It was started by a dozen 12–15 year-old kids from Blackstone Avenue in Woodlawn.
4. At this time, grammar or elementary school consisted of grades one through eight.
5. High school fraternities were not sanctioned by the authorities, as they had no legal standing.
6. The drugstore was located at 65th Street and Ellis and owned by Nathan Sarnat, Israel's son. Bernie worked at that drugstore after the one owned by his father at 69th and Indiana had been sold and until his father purchased the drugstore at 57th and Blackstone Ave.

Chapter 16. Undergraduate School Years (1929–1933)

1. Jean Block *Houses in Hyde Park*, University of Chicago Press (1978).
2. The only exceptions were the period of 1936–1937 in Los Angeles and 1940–1941 at Cook County Hospital in Chicago.
3. Sidney Smith went on to do early work on heart valves and the artificial heart.

Chapter 18. University of Illinois (1937–1940)

1. With the Gies' report of 1926 (which brought dental schools up to date from commercial institutions to university affiliated institutions), the Chicago College of Dental Surgery began to be associated with Loyola University until the dental school was finally closed in 1993.
2. Doctor Black was the son of G. V. Black (1836–1915) who was also a dean as well as a founder of the dental school at Northwestern. Although he was self-educated, G. V. Black was a pioneer in modern dentistry whose accomplishments ranged from bacteriology to patient care. When he died in 1915, Black held professorships in dental pathology, bacteriology and operative dentistry, and served as dean of Northwestern University Dental School, which graduated its last dental class in 2001.
3. Dr. Louis Reif and Dr. Schour had been high school classmates together. It was also Louis Reif who initially recommended that Jack, Bernie's older brother, study dentistry.
4. Sarnat, B. G. The teeth as permanent chronologic recorders of systemic disease: A clinical and experimental study of enamel hypoplasia. *Proc. Inst. Med. Chicago.* **13**:114–116 (1940).
5. Adams, C. O and Sarnat, B. G. Effects of yellow phosphorus and arsenic trioxide in growing bones and growing teeth. *Arch. Path.* **30**:1192–1202 (1940).
6. Sarnat B. G. and Hook, W. E. Effect of hibernation on rate of eruption and dentin apposition in the ground squirrel incisor. *Proc. Exp. Biol. Med.* **46**:685–688 (1941). Reprinted *Anat. Rec.* **83**:471–493 (1942).

7. Schour, I., Hoffman, M. M. Sarnat B. G. and Engel, M. B. Vital staining of growing bones and teeth with alizarine red S. *J. Dent. Res.* **20**:411–418 (1941).

8. Sarnat, B. G. Schour I. and Heupel, R. Roentgenographic diagnosis of congenital syphilis. *J. Am. Med. Assoc.* **116**:2745–2747 (1941).

9. Sarnat B. G. and Shaw, N. G. Dental development in congenital syphilis. *Am. J. Dis. Child.* **64**:771–788 (1942).

10. Occupational disease was concerned with exposure to lead, arsenic, and bismuth, heavy metals used in the preparation of war materials.

11. Schour I. and Sarnat, B. G. Oral manifestations of occupational origin. *J. Am. Med. Assoc.* **120**:1197–1207 (1942).

12. Schour I. and Sarnat, B. G. Oral occupational diseases. Dentistry, *A Digest of Pract.* **3**:4 page insert (1942).

13. This Great Lakes shipping line was known colloquially, as the 'C & B'.

14. Besides being an Irish-Catholic, the actual identity of the stoker was unknown. The shipping line asked few questions, they hired anyone who was willing to work the long and exhausting hours for little pay.

Chapter 19. Marriage to Rhoda E. Gerard

1. Encyclopedia Judaica, Vol. 7, p. 551.

2. In 1917, at the instigation of one of the firms for which he acted as consultant during WW1, he changed his surname from Gesundheit to Gerard as the former was seen as too Germanic.

3. His degree was actually from the Mason Science College, which was one of the colleges that was a forerunner of the University of Birmingham. The University of Birmingham was officially founded in 1900.

4. Ellis Island was initially opened in 1892 but a fire completely destroyed the building in June 1897. It opened for business again on Dec. 17, 1900.

5. Gerard, Graham & Co. *Professional Policies and Practices*, 1921, an in-house document. The company specialized in industrial engineering. They provided consulting on a wide range of problems, ranging from layout of the physical plant, inventory, purchasing, cost control, sales policies, wages, executive management, time studies, etc.

He was ahead of his time in many areas (e.g., see Thomas Friedman, *The World is Flat*, 2005).

6. This same Benjamin Graham was secretary at Gerard, Graham & Co., as well as the teacher and mentor of Warren Buffett. ·

7. In about that late 1980's Bernie had a graduate student from the same Swiss region. He told Bernie that the school had been sold and the building was now occupied by an insurance company.

8. A sum that was probably equivalent to about $1,185,000 in 2002 dollars.

9. Stenotyping came in very handy later in taking notes at UCLA and to this day.

Chapter 20. Training in Plastic and Reconstructive Surgery (1941–1946)

1. ENT, Ear, Nose and Throat.

2. Surgery of the nose and nasal passages.

3. Alizarin red S is a biological stain used to detect the presence of calcium, among other elements, in bone tissue.

4. Blair, V. P. and Byars, L. T. (with credit to Sarnat, B. G. in a footnote). Hits, strikes and outs in the use of pedicle flaps for nasal restoration or correction. *Surg. Gynecol. Obstet.* **82**:367 (1946).

5. Randall, P., McCarthy, J. G. and Wray, R. E. History of the American Association of Plastic Surgeons, 1921 to 1996. *Plast. Reconstr. Surg.* **97**:1254 (1996).

6. Stelnicki E. J., Young, V. L., Francel, T. and Randall, P. Vilray P. Blair, his surgical descendants, and their roles in plastic surgery development. *Plast. Reconstr. Surg.* **103**:1990–2009 (1999).

7. Byars, L. T. and Sarnat, B. G. Congenital macrogingivae (fibroniatosis gingivae) and hypertrichosis. *Surgery* **15**:34 (1944).

8. Byars. L. T. and Sarnat. B. G. Surgery of the mandible: The ameloblastoma. *Surg. Gynecol. Obstet.* **81**:575 (1945).

9. Byars, L. T. and Sarnat, B. G. Surgery of the mandible: The ameloblastoma. (Reprint). *Am. J. Orth. Oral. Surg.* **32**:34 (1946).

10. Byars. L. T. and Sarnat, B. G. Mandibular tumors: A clinical, roentgenographic and histopathologic study. *Surg. Gynecol. Obstet.* **83**:355 (1946).

11. Sarnat, B. G. and Laskin, D. M. *Diagnosis and Surgical Management of Diseases of the Temporomandibular Joint.* Charles C Thomas, Springfield, Illinois (1962).
12. Sarnat, B. G. and Greeley, P. Effect, of injury upon growth and some comments on surgical treatment. *Plast. Reconstr. Surg.* 11:39 (1953).

Chapter 21. Life in St. Louis and Chicago

1. This was a payment closer to perhaps $6,000 in today's dollars. It was common practice in Chicago at that time.

Chapter 22. Practice of Plastic Surgery (1946–1956)

1. Material here is adapted from the American Board of Plastic Surgeons, Inc. (2004).

Chapter 23. Professor of Oral and Maxillofacial Surgery and Plastic Surgery (1946–1956)

1. Sarnat, B. G. and Engel, M. B. 1951. A serial study of mandibular growth after removal of the condyle in the Macaca rhesus monkey. *Plast. Reconstr. Surg.* 7:364–380 (1950).
2. Gans, B. J. and Sarnat, B. G. Sutural facial growth of the Macaca rhesus monkey: A gross and serial roentgenographic study by means of metallic implants. *Am. J. Orthodont.* 37:827–841 (1951).
3. Selman, A. J. and Sarnat, B. G. A Headholder for Serial Roentgenography of the Rabbit Skull. *Anat. Rec.* 115:627–634 (1953).
4. Rosen, M. D. and Sarnat, B. G. A comparison of the volume of the left and right maxillary sinuses in dogs. *Anat. Rec.* 120:65–72 (1954).
5. Robinson, I. B. and Sarnat, B. G. Growth pattern of the pig mandible: A serial roentgenographic study using metallic implants. *Am. J. Anat.* 96:37–64 (1955).

6. Rosen, M. D. and Sarnat, B. G. Change of volume of the maxillary sinus of the dog after extraction of adjacent teeth. *Oral Surg. Oral Med. and Oral Path.* **8**:420–429 (1955).

7. Selman, A. J. and Sarnat, B. G. Sutural bone growth of the rabbit snout: A gross and serial roentgenographic study by means of metallic implants. *Am. J. Anat.* **97**:395–408 (1955).

8. Roy, E. W. and Sarnat, B. G. Growth in length of rabbit ribs at the costochondral junction. *Surg. Gyn. Obst.* **103**:481–486 (1956).

9. Sarnat, B. G. Facial and neurocranial growth after removal of the mandibular condyle in the Macaca rhesus monkey. *Am. J. Surg.* **94**:19–30 (1957).

10. Selman, A. J. and Sarnat, B. G. Growth of the rabbit snout after extirpation of the frontonasal suture: A gross and serial roentgenographic study by means of metallic implants. *Am. J. Anat.* **101**:273–293 (1957).

11. Sarnat, B. G. Palatal and facial growth in Macaca rhesus monkeys with surgically produced palatal clefts. *Plast. Reconstr. Surg.* **22**:29–41 (1958).

12. Sarnat, B. G. (ed.). *The Temporomandibular Joint.* Charles C Thomas Publisher, Springfield (1951).

13. Sarnat, B. G. and Laskin, D. M. Surgery of the temporomandibular joint. Chap. 10, in *The Temporomandibular Joint* (B. G. Sarnat, ed.). Charles C Thomas, Publisher, Springfield, Illinois, 2nd ed. (1964).

14. Sarnat, B. G. and Laskin, D. M. (eds.). *The Temporomandibular Joint: A Biological Basis for Clinical Practice*, 3rd ed., Charles C Thomas, Publisher, Springfield, Illinois (1980).

15. Sarnat, B. G. and Laskin, D. M. *The Temporomandibular Joint: A Biological Basis for Clinical Practice* (3rd Edition). Translated into Japanese, Yojiro Kawamura, Ishiyaka, Pub. Tokyo, Japan (1983).

16. Sarnat, B. G. and Laskin, D. M. (eds.). *The Temporomandibular Joint: A Biological Basis for Clinical Practice*, 4th ed., W.B, Saunders, Publisher, Philadelphia, Pennsylvania (1991).

17. Gray's Anatomy, P. 402, 26th ed. (1954).

18. Sarnat, B. G. *Current Advances in Dentistry.* Contributor and Editor of section on Oral Diagnosis and Cancer Control. University of Illinois Press (1949)

19. Sarnat, B. G. Cancer in childhood. *Your Child Patient* **1**:10–14 (1950).

20. Sarnat, B. G. and Schour, I. *Oral and Facial Cancer*. The Year Book Publishers, Inc., Chicago (1950).

21. Sarnat, B. G. *Current Advances in Dentistry*. Chart on Oral and Facial Examination. Adapted from Sarnat and Schour, *Oral and Facial Cancer*. The Year Book Publishers, Inc. University of Illinois Press, Chicago (1950).

22. Sarnat, B. G. and Schour, I. Oral and facial cancer. *General Pract.* **3**:41–51 (1951).

23. Sarnat, B. G. and Schour, I., Medichrome Series 35 mm Slides (188). Clay-Adams Company Inc., New York (1952).

24. Sarnat, B. G. and Schour, I. *Oral and Facial Cancer*. The Year Book Publishers, Inc., Chicago. Reprinted (1953).

25. Sarnat, B. G. and Schour, I. Oral and facial cancer. *Dental Radiog. and Photog.* **27**:1–6, 14–16 (1954).

26. Sarnat, B. G. and Schour, I. Oral and facial cancer. *N. Y. State Dent. J.* **20**:267–270 (1954).

27. Sarnat, B. G. and Schour, I. *Mund- und Gesichts-Krebs. Die Quintessenz.* **8**:1–6 (1954).

28. Sarnat, B. G. and Schour, I. *Cancer Da Face E Da Boca*. Translated into Portuguese by Claudio Mello, Editoria Cientifica, Publishers, Rio de Janiero. (1956).

29. Sarnat, B. G. and Schour, I. *Essentials of Oral and Facial Cancer*, 2nd ed., The Year Book Publishers Inc., Chicago (1957).

30. Sarnat, B. G. *Current Advances in Dentistry*. Contributor and Editor of section on Diseases of the Mouth. University of Illinois Press (1950).

31. Sarnat, B. G. *Current Advances in Dentistry*. Contributor and Editor of section on The Denture and the Temporomandibular Joint. University of Illinois Press (1951).

32. Sarnat, B. G. *Current Advances in Dentistry*. Surgical Treatment of Malocclusion in section on Normal and Abnormal Occlusion. University of Illinois Press (1951).

33. Sarnat, B. G. *Current Advance in Dentistry*. Contributor to Section on Developmental Anomalies in Dental Practice. University of Illinois Press (1952).

34. Sarnat, B. G. *Current Advances in Dentistry*. Editor of Section on Emergency Problems in Dental Practice and contributor (Facial Fractures). University of Illinois Press (1954).

Chapter 26. Foreign Travel

1. Sarnat, B. G. Differential effect of surgical trauma to the nasal bones and septum upon rabbit snout growth. *Trans. 4th Int. Cong. Plast. Surg.* Publisher: Excerpta Medica Foundation, Amsterdam **66**:38–43 (1969).

Chapter 27. A Close Brush with Death

1. The eventual sale of the home was delayed until 1972 and took place under totally different circumstances.
2. Sarnat, B. G., Kaplan, L. and Barshop, N. Thirty-seven year postoperative, postchemotherapy follow-up of "Dukes" C Carcinoma of the colon with no recurrence. *Digestive Dis. Sci.* **43**:1672–1674 (1998).

Chapter 29. Academia and Research (1956–Present)

1. Sarnat, B. G. Healing of unrepaired surgical cleft palate in the Macaca rhesus monkey. *Cleft Palate Bull.* **8**:11–12 (1958).
2. Sarnat, B. G. and Robinson, I. B. Growth of the mandible: Some experimental and clinical considerations. *J. South. Calif. S.D.A.* **28**:354–364 (1960).
3. Wexler, M. R. and Sarnat, B. G. Rabbit snout growth: Effect of injury to the septovomeral region. *Arch. Otolaryn.* **74**:305–313 (1961).
4. Sarnat, B. G. and Laskin, D. M. *Diagnosis and Surgical Management of Diseases of the Temporomandibular Joint.* Charles C Thomas, Publisher, Springfield, Illinois (1962).
5. Sarnat, B. G. Facial plastic surgery. Chap. 6. In: E. Epstein (ed.). *Skin Surgery.* Lea and Febiger, Publisher, Philadelphia, 2nd Edition (1962).
6. Herzberg, F. and Sarnat, B. G. Radiographic changes in the bony trabecular pattern in the mandible of growing Macaca rhesus monkeys following condylar resection. *Anat. Rec.* **144**:129–134 (1962).

7. Wexler, M. R., and Sarnat, B. G. Rabbit snout growth: Effect of injury to the septovomeral region. *Arch. Otolaryn.* **74**:305–313 (1961).

8. Wexler, M. R. and Sarnat, B. G. Rabbit snout growth after dislocation of nasal septum. *Arch. Otolaryn.* **81**:68–71 (1965).

9. Sarnat, B. G. and Wexler, M. R. Growth of the face and jaws after resection of the septal cartilage in the rabbit. *Am. J. Anat.* **118**:755–767 (1966).

10. Sarnat, B. G. and Wexler, M. R. Rabbit snout growth after resection of central linear segments of nasal septal cartilage. *Acta Otolaryn.* **63**:467–478 (1967).

11. Sarnat, B. G. and Wexler, M. R. The snout after resection of nasal · septum in adult rabbits. *Arch. Otolaryn.* **86**:463–466 (1967).

12. Sarnat, B. G. and Wexler, M. R. Postnatal growth of the nose and face after resection of septal cartilage in the rabbit. *Oral Surg. Oral Med. Oral Path.* **26**:712–727 (1968).

13. Sarnat, B. G. and Wexler, M. R. Longitudinal development of upper facial deformity after septal resection in growing rabbits. *Brit. J. Plast. Surg.* **22**:313–323 (1969).

14. Sarnat, B. G. and Muchnic, H. Facial changes after mandibular condylectomy in growing and adult monkeys. *J. Dent. Res. Abstr.* **89** (1970).

15. Sarnat, B. G. and Muchnic, H. Facial skeletal changes after mandibular condylectomy in the adult monkey. *J. Anat.* **108**:323–338 (1971).

16. Sarnat, B. G. and Muchnic, H. Facial Skeletal changes after mandibular condylectomy in growing and adult monkeys. *Am. J. Orthod.* **60**:33–45 (1971).

17. Sarnat, B. G. and Selman, A. Growth pattern of the nasal bone region in the rabbit. *J. Dent. Res.* **56**:352 (1977).

18. Sarnat, B. G. and Selman, A. J. Growth pattern of the rabbit snout dorsum: A serial cephalometric radiographic study with radiopaque implants. *J. Anat.* **124**(2):469–474 (1977).

19. Sarnat, B G. and Selman, A. J. Growth pattern of the rabbit nasal bone region. A combined serial gross and radiographic study with metallic implants. *Acta Anat.* **101**:193–201 (1978).

20. Sarnat, B. G. and Selman, A. J. Growth pattern of the rabbit nasal bone region. *Rhinology* **20**:93–105 (1982).

21. Sarnat, B. G. and Shanedling, P. D. Postnatal growth of the upper face and orbit. *J. Dent. Res.* **43**:756–757 (1964).
22. Sarnat, B. G. and Shanedling, P. D. Postnatal growth of the orbit and upper face in rabbits after exenteration of the orbit. *Arch. Ophthal.* **13**: 829–837 (1965).
23. Sarnat, B. G. and Shanedling, P. D. Orbital volume following evisceration, enucleation and exenteration in rabbits. *Am. J. Ophthal.* **70**:787–799 (1970).
24. Sarnat, B. G. and Shanedling, P. D. Orbital growth after evisceration or enucleation without and with implants. *J. Dent. Res.* Abstr. **98** (1971).
25. Sarnat, B. G. and Shanedling, P. D. Orbital growth after evisceration or enucleation without and with implants. *Acta Anat.* **82**:497–511 (1972).
26. Sarnat, B. G. and Shanedling, P. D. Orbital volume after periodic intrabular injections of silicone in growing rabbits. *J. Dent. Res.* **52**:280 (1973).
27. Gault, I. G. and Sarnat, B. G. Permanent duplication of the freshly enucleated rabbit eye. *Ophthalmologica* **168**:154–159 (1974).
28. Petrula, D. and Sarnat, B. G. Comparison of linear and volumetric measurements of the rabbit orbit. *Ophthalmic Res.* **6**:43–54 (1974).
29. Sarnat, B. G. and Shanedling, P. D. Increased orbital volume after periodic intrabular injections of silicone in growing rabbits. *Am. J. Anat.* **140**:523–532 (1974).
30. Sarnat, B. G. Adult rabbit eye and orbital volumes after periodic intrabulbar injections of silicone. *Ophthalmologica* **178**:43–48 (1979).
31. Sarnat, B. G. Eye volume in young and adult rabbits, *Acta Anat.* **106**:462–467 (1980).
32. Sarnat, B. G. Orbital volume in young and adult rabbits, *Anat. Embryol.* **159**:211–221 (1980).
33. Alexandridis, C. and Sarnat, B. G. Comparison of gravimetric and linear methods to determine rabbit eye volume. *Ophthalmic Res.* **12**:240–243 (1980).
34. Sarnat, B. G. Eye and orbital size in the young and adult. Some postnatal experimental and clinical relationships. *Ophthalmologica* **185**:74–89 (1982).

35. Lestrel, P. E., Sarnat, B. G., Read, D. W., Wolfe, C. A. and Bodt, A. Three-dimensional characterization of eye orbit shape: Fourier descriptors. *Am. J. Phys. Anthrop. Suppl.* **16**:134 (1993).

36. Lestrel, P. E., Wolfe, C. A., Read, D. W. and Sarnat, B. G. A numerical analysis of the rabbit orbital margin: Three-dimensional fourier descriptors. *J. Dent. Res.* **74**:580 (1995).

37. Long, R., Greulich, R. C. and Sarnat, B. G. Regional variations in chondrocyte proliferation in the cartilaginous nasal septum of the growing rabbit. *J. Dent. Res.* **47**:137 (1968).

38. Long, R., Greulich, R. C. and Sarnat, B. G. Regional variations in chondrocyte proliferation in the cartilaginous nasal septum of the growing rabbit. *J. Dent. Res.* **47**:505 (1968).

39. Prechter, T. K. and Sarnat, B. G. Comparison of direct and indirect determinations of rabbit orbital volume. *Acta Morphol. Neerl-Scand.* **11**: 151–160 (1973).

40. Sarnat, B. G., McNabb, E. and Glass, M. Craniofacial growth: I. Turtle shell growth in a controlled laboratory environment. *J. Dent. Res.* **58**:148 (1979).

41. Sarnat, B. G. and McNabb, E. G. Sutural bone growth of the Turtle *Chrysemys scripta* plastron. *J. Dent. Res.* **60**:579 (1981).

42. Sarnat, B. G., Feigenbaum, J. A., Trieger, N. and Herzberg, F. Adult monkey face after resection of trigeminal nerve motor branch. *J. Dent. Res.* **54**:163 (1975).

43. Sarnat, B. G., Feigenbaum, J. A. and Krogman, W. M. Adult monkey coronoid process after resection of trigeminal nerve motor root. *Am. J. Anat.* **150**:129–138 (1977).

44. Sarnat, B. G., McNabb, E. G. and Glass, M. Growth of the Turtle *Chrysemys scripta* under constant controlled laboratory conditions. *Anat. Rec.* **199**: 433–439 (1981).

45. Lestrel, P. E., Sarnat, B. G. and McNabb, E. G. Fourier analysis of carapace shape: Growth of the Turtle *Chrysemys scripta*. *J. Dent. Res.* **66**: 347 (1987).

46. Lestrel, P. E., Sarnat, B. G. and McNabb, E. G. Carapace growth of the Turtle *Chrysemys scripta*: A longitudinal study of shape using fourier analysis. *Anat. Anz.* (Jena) **168**: 135–143 (1989).

47. Dixon, A. D. and Sarnat, B. G. (eds.). *Factors and Mechanisms Influencing Bone Growth.* Alan R. Liss, Inc. Publisher, New York (1982).

48. Dixon, A. D. and Sarnat, B. G. (eds.). *Normal and Abnormal Bone Growth: Basic and Clinical Research*. Alan R. Liss, Inc. Publisher, New York (1985).

49. Dixon, A. D., Sarnat, B. G. and Hoyte, D. A. N. (eds.). *Fundamentals of Bone Growth: Methodology and Applications*. CRC Press Inc. Publisher, Boca Raton (1991).

50. Sarnat, B. G. and Laskin, D. M. (eds.). *The Temporomandibular Joint: A Biological Basis for Clinical Practice*, 3rd ed., Charles C Thomas, Publisher, Springfield, (1980).

51. Laskin, D. M. and Sarnat, B. G. History and Physical Examination In *The Temporomandibular Joint: A Biological Basis for Clinical Practice*. W.B, Saunders, Pub. Philadelphia, 4th Edition (1991).

52. Sarnat, B. G. and Laskin, D. M. *The Temporomandibular Joint: A Biological Basis for Clinical Practice* (3rd Edition). Translated into Japanese, Yojiro Kawamura, reviewer, Ishiyaka, Pub., Tokyo (1983).

53. Sarnat, B. G. and Schour, I. *Cancer Da Face E Da Boca*. Translated into Portuguese by Claudio Mello, Editoria Cientifica, Publishers, Rio de Janiero (1956).

54. Adams, C. O. and Sarnat, B. G. Effects of yellow phosphorus and arsenic trioxide on growing bones and growing teeth. *Arch. Path.* **30**:1192–1202 (1940).

55. Sarnat, B. G. and Hook, W. E. Effect of hibernation on rate of eruption and dentin apposition in the ground squirrel incisor. *Proc. Soc. Exp. Biol. Med.* **46**:685–688 (1941).

56. Schour, I., Hoffman, M. H., Sarnat, B. G. and Engel, M. B. Vital staining of growing bones and teeth with alizarine red S. *J. Dent. Res.* **20**:411–418 (1941).

57. Sarnat, B. G. and Hook W. E. Effects of hibernation on tooth development. *Anat. Rec.* **83**:471–493 (1942).

58. Gans, B. J. and Sarnat, B. G. Sutural facial growth of the Macaca rhesus monkey: A gross and serial roentgenographic study by means of metallic implants. *Am. J. Orthod.* **37**:827–841 (1951).

59. Robinson, I. B. and Sarnat, B. G. Growth pattern of the pig mandible: A serial roentgenographic study using metallic implants. *Am. J. Anat.* **96**:37–64 (1955).

60. Selman, A. J. and Sarnat, B. G. Sutural bone growth of the rabbit snout: A gross and serial roentgenographic study by means of metallic implants. *Am. J. Anat.* **97**:395–408 (1955).

61. Sarnat, B. G. and Hook W. E. Effects of hibernation on tooth development. *Anat. Rec.* **83**:471–493 (1942).

62. Sarnat, B. G. Oral-Plastic Surgery. Chap. 5, In *Skin Surgery* (E. Epstein, ed.). Lea and Febiger, Publisher, Philadelphia (1956).

63. Sarnat, B. G. Facial and neurocranial growth after removal of the mandibular condyle in the Macaca rhesus monkey. *Am. J. Surg.* **94**:19–30 (1957).

64. Sarnat, B. G. Palatal and facial growth in Macaca rhesus monkeys with surgically produced palatal clefts. *Plast. Reconstr. Surg.* **22**:29–41 (1958).

65. Sarnat, B. G. Gross growth and regrowth of sutures: Reflections on some personal research. *J. Craniofac. Surg.* **14**:438–444 (2003).

66. Long, R., Greulich, R. C. and Sarnat, B. G. Regional variations in chondrocyte proliferation in the cartilaginous nasal septum of the growing rabbit. *J. Dent. Res.* **47**:505 (1968).

67. Sarnat, B. G. The imprint method to determine orbital volume in the rabbit. *Ophthalmologica* **160**:142–151 (1970).

68. Selman, A. J. and Sarnat, B. G. Growth of the rabbit snout after extirpation of the frontonasal suture: A gross and serial roentgenographic study by means of metallic implants. *Am. J. Anat.* **101**:273–293 (1957).

69. Sarnat, B. G. and Selman, A. J. Growth Pattern of the rabbit nasal bone region. A combined serial gross and radiographic study with metallic implants. *Acta Anat.* **101**:193–201 (1978).

70. Wexler, M. R. and Sarnat, B. G. Rabbit snout growth: Effect of injury to the septovomeral region. *Arch. Otolaryn.* **74**:305–313 (1961).

71. Sarnat, B. G. and Schour, I. Enamel hypoplasia (Chronologic Enamel Aplasia) in relation to systemic disease: A chronologic, morphologic and etiologic classification. Part I. J.A.D.A. **28**:1989–2000, (December 1941).

72. Sarnat, B. G. and Schour, I. Enamel hypoplasia (Chronologic Enamel Aplasia) in relation, to systemic disease: A chronologic,

morphologic and etiologic classification, Part II. J.A.D.A. **29**:67–75 (January 1942).

73. Sarnat, B. G., Schour, I. and Heupel, R. Roentgenographic diagnosis of congenital syphilis. J.A.M.A. **116**:2745–2747 (June 1941).

74. Sarnat, B. G. and Shaw, N. G. Dental development in congenital syphilis. *Am. J. Dis. Child.* **64**:771–788 (1942).

75. Sarnat, B. G., Brodie, A. G. and Kubacki, W. H. A fourteen year report of facial growth in case of complete anodontia with ectodermal dysplasia. *Am. J. Dis. Child.* **86**:162–169 (1953).

76. Robinson, I. B. and Sarnat, B. G. Roentgen studies of the maxillae and mandible in sickle-cell anemia. *Radiology* **58**:517–523 (1952).

77. Sarnat, B. G. and Schour, I. *Oral and Facial Cancer.* The Year Book Publishers, Inc., Chicago (1950).

78. Sarnat, B. G. and Schour, I. *Oral and Facial Cancer.* The Year Book Publishers, Inc., Chicago, Reprint (1953).

79. Sarnat, B. G. and Schour, I. *Essentials of Oral and Facial Cancer,* 2nd ed. The Year Book Publishers Inc., Chicago (1957).

80. Sarnat, B. G. (ed.). *The Temporomandibular Joint.* Charles C Thomas Pub., Springfield, (1951).

81. Sarnat, B. G. (ed.). *The Temporomandibular Joint,* 2nd ed. Charles C Thomas, Pub., Springfield (1964).

82. Sarnat, B. G. and Laskin, D. M. (eds.). *The Temporomandibular Joint: A Biological Basis for Clinical Practice,* 3rd ed. Charles C Thomas, Publisher, Springfield (1980).

83. Laskin, D. M. and Sarnat, B. G. History and Physical Examination In *The Temporomandibular Joint: A Biological Basis for Clinical Practice,* 4th ed. W. B. Saunders, Publisher, Philadelphia (1991).

Chapter 31. A Day in the Life of a Biological Scientist

1. Sarnat, B. G. The teeth as permanent chronologic recorders of systemic disease: A clinical and experimental study of enamel hypoplasia. *Proc. Inst. Med. Chicago* **13**:114. Reprinted from University of Illinois *College of Dent. Bull.* **23**:5 (1940).

2. Sarnat, B. G. and Shaw, N. G. Dental development in congenital syphilis. Reprinted *Am. J. Orthod. Oral Surg.* **29**:270–284 (1943).

3. Sarnat, B. G. Effect of systemic disease on growing teeth. *Proc. Inst. of Med., Chicago* **13**:368–369 (1941).

4. Gans, B. J. and Sarnat, B. G. Sutural facial growth of the Macaca rhesus monkey: A gross and serial roentgenographic study by means of metallic implants. *Am. J. Orthodont.* **37**:827–841 (1951).

5. Laskin, D. M., Sarnat, B. G. and Bain, J. A. Respiration and anaerobic glycolysis of transplanted cartilage, *Proc. Soc. Exp. Biol. Med.* **19**:474–476 (1952).

6. Laskin, D. M. and Sarnat, B. G. The metabolism of fresh, transplanted and preserved cartilage. *Surg. Gyn Obst.* **96**:493–499 (1953).

7. Selman, A. J. and Sarnat, B. G. A headholder for serial roentgenography of the rabbit skull. *Anat. Rec.* **115**:627–634 (1953).

8. Rosen, M. D. and Sarnat, B. G. A comparison of the volume of the left and right maxillary sinuses in dogs. *Anat. Rec.* **120**:65–72 (1954).

9. Sarnat, B. G. and Laskin D. M. Cartilage and cartilage implants. Collective Reviews Section, *Int. Abstr. Surg. Gyn. Obst.* **99**:521–541 (1954).

10. Akamine, R. N., Engel, M. B. and Sarnat B. G. Histochemical studies of cartilage implants. *J. Bone Joint Surg.* **32**-A:1166–1174 (1954).

11. Robinson, I. B. and Sarnat, B. G. Growth pattern of the pig mandible: A serial roentgenographic study using metallic implants. *Am. J. Anat.* **96**:37–64 (1955).

12. Rosen, M. D. and Sarnat, B. G. Change of volume of the maxillary sinus of the dog after extraction of adjacent teeth. *Oral Surg. Oral Med. Oral Path.* **8**:420–429 (1955).

13. Selman, A. J. and Sarnat, B. G. Sutural bone growth of the rabbit snout: A gross and serial roentgenographic study by means of metallic implants. *Am. J. Anat.* **97**:395–408 (1955).

14. Roy, E. W. and Sarnat, B. G. Growth in length of rabbit ribs at the costochondral junction. *Surg. Gyn. Obst.* **103**:481–486 (1956).

15. Selman, A. J. and Sarnat, B. G. Growth of the rabbit snout after extirpation of the frontonasal suture: A gross and serial roentgenographic study by means of metallic implants. *Am. J. Anat.* **101**: 273–293 (1957).

16. Pruzansky, S., Ricketts, R., Sarnat, B. G. and Engel, M. B. Cephalometric, electromyographic and laminagraphic analysis of two cases of bilateral subcondylar osteotomy. *Am. J. Orthod.* **37**:147 (1951).

17. Sarnat, B. G. and Engel, M. B. A serial study of mandibular growth after removal of the condyle in the Macaca rhesus monkey. *Plast. Reconstr. Surg.* **7**:364–380 (1951).

18. Sarnat, B. G. and Greeley, P. W. Effect of injury upon growth and some comments on surgical treatment. *Plast. Reconstr. Surg.* **11**:39–48 (1953).

19. Sarnat, B. G. Brodie, A. G. and Kubacki, W. H. A fourteen year report of facial growth in case of complete anodontia with ectodermal dysplasia. *Am. J. Dis. Child.* **86**:162–169 (1953).

20. Weinmann, J. P., Sarnat, B. G. and Sicher, H. Tissue reaction in surgical defects of the palate in the Macaca rhesus. *Oral Surg. Oral Med. Oral Path.* **11**:20–25 (1958).

21. Wexler, M. R. and Sarnat, B. G. Rabbit snout growth: Effect of injury to the septovomeral region. *Arch. Otolaryn.* **74**:305–313 (1961).

22. Wexler, M. R. and Sarnat, B. G. Rabbit snout growth after dislocation of nasal septum. *Arch. Otolaryn.* **81**:68–71 (1965).

23. Sarnat, B. G. and Shanedling, P. D. Postnatal growth of the orbit and upper face in rabbits after exenteration of the orbit. *Arch. Ophthal.* **13**:829–837 (1965).

24. Sarnat, B. G. and Wexler, M. R. Growth of the face and jaws after resection of the septal cartilage in the rabbit. *Am. J. Anat.* **118**:755–767 (1966).

25. Sarnat, B. G. and Wexler, M. R. The snout after resection of nasal septum in adult rabbits. *Arch. Otolaryn.* **86**:463–466 (1967).

26. Long, R., Greulich, R. C. and Sarnat, B. G. Regional variations in chondrocyte proliferation in the cartilaginous nasal septum of the growing rabbit. *J. Dent. Res.* **47**:505 (1968).

27. Sarnat, B. G. and Wexler, M. R. Longitudinal development of upper facial deformity after septal resection in growing rabbits. *Brit. J. Plastic Surg.* **22**:313–323 (1969).

28. Sarnat, B. G. The imprint method to determine orbital volume in the rabbit. *Ophthalmologica* **160**:142–151 (1970).

29 Sarnat, B. G. and Shanedling, P. D. Orbital volume following evisceration, enucleation and exenteration in Rabbits. *Am. J. Ophthalm.* **70**:787–799 (1970).

30. Sarnat, B. G. and Muchnic, H. Facial skeletal changes after mandibular condylectomy in the adult monkey. *J. Anat.* **108**:323–338 (1971).

31. Sarnat, B. G. and Shanedling, P. D. Increased orbital volume after periodic intrabular injections of silicone in growing rabbits. *Am J. Anat.* **140**:523–532 (1974).

32. Sarnat, B. G., Feigenbaum, J. A. and Krogman, W. M. Adult monkey coronoid process after resection of trigeminal nerve motor root. *Am. J. Anat.* **150**:129–138 (1977).

33. Sarnat, B. G., McNabb, E. G. and Glass, M. Growth of the Turtle *Chrysemys scripta* under constant controlled laboratory conditions. *Anat. Rec.* **199**:433–439 (1981).

34. Sarnat, B. G. and McNabb, E. G. Sutural bone growth of the Turtle *Chrysemys scripta* plastron: A serial radiographic study by means of radiopaque implants. *Growth* **45**:123–134 (1981).

35. Robinson, I. B. and Sarnat, B. G. Growth pattern of the pig mandible: A serial roentgenographic study using metallic implants. *Am. J. Anat.* **96**:37–64 (1955).

36. Sarnat, B. G. and Selman, A. Growth pattern of the rabbit nasal bone region. A combined serial gross and radiographic study with metallic implants. *Acta Anat.* **101**:193–201 (1978).

37. Gans, B. J. and Sarnat, B. G. Sutural facial growth of the Macaca rhesus monkey: A gross and serial roentgenographic study by means of metallic implants *Am. J. Orthod.* **37**:827–841 (1951).

38. Selman, A. J. and Sarnat, B. G. Growth of the rabbit snout after extirpation of the frontonasal suture: A gross and serial roentgenographic study by means of metallic implants. *Am. J. Anat.* **101**(2):273–293 (1957).

39. Sarnat, B. G. and Engel, M. B. A serial study of mandibular growth after removal of the condyle in the Macaca rhesus monkey. *Plast. Reconstr. Surg.* **7**:364–380 (1951).

40. Sarnat, B. G. Facial and neurocranial growth after removal of the mandibular condyle in the Macaca rhesus monkey. *Am. J. Surg.* **94**:19–30 (1957).

41. Sarnat, B. G. and Muchnic, H. Facial skeletal changes after mandibular condylectomy in the adult monkey. *J. Anat.* **108**:323–338 (1971).

42. Sarnat, B. G. and Selman, A. J. Growth pattern of the rabbit nasal bone region. *Rhinology* **20**:93–105 (1982).

43. Selman, A. J. and Sarnat, B. G. Sutural bone growth of the rabbit snout: A gross and serial roentgenographic study by means of metallic implants. *Am. J. Anat.* **97**:395–408 (1955).

44. Sarnat, B. G. and Selman, A. Growth pattern of the rabbit nasal bone region. A combined serial gross and radiographic study with metallic implants. *Acta Anat.* **101**:193–201 (1978).

45. Lestrel, P. E., Sarnat, B. G. and McNabb, E. G. Carapace growth of the Turtle *Chrysemys scripta*: A longitudinal study of shape using fourier analysis. *Anat. Anz.* (Jena) **168**:135–143 (1989).

CHRONOLOGY

Notes

1. The material in this section was developed with the assistance of: A guide to the 20th century. http://www.channel4.com/history/microsites/H/history/guide20/part01.html Retrieved May 27, 2007.
2. The material with highlighted borders refers to events dealing directly with Bernie Sarnat's personal and professional life.

1878	Birth of Bernie's father, Isadore Sarnatzky in Skidel, Belarus
1880	Birth of Bernie's mother, Fanny Sidran Silverman in Volkovysk

1881	First pogroms against Russian Jews leading thousands to emigrate
1894	Rule of Tsar Nicholas II begins (executed by Bolsheviks in 1918)
1899	Beginning of Boer War (ended in 1902)
1900	Sigmund Freud publishes *The Interpretation of Dreams* Quantum physics established by Max Planck
1901	Death of Queen Victoria President William McKinley is assassinated

	Marriage of Isadore and Fanny Sarnatzky, Bernie's parents
1902	Birth of Jacob, Isadore's and Fanny's first son
1903	First powered flight at Kitty Hawk, NC by Wilbur and Orville Wright Pogroms against Russian Jews intensified (continued until 1906)
1904	Russo-Japanese War (ended in 1905 with a defeat for Russia)
	Birth of Tena, Isadore's and Fanny's daughter
1905	Special Theory of Relativity published by Albert Einstein
1906	San Francisco earthquake with 1,000 dead and 200,000 homeless
1907	Isadore Sarnatzky migrates to the United States, followed by Fanny in 1909 with their two young children, Jacob and Tena
1908	Israel Sarnatzky, Bernie's uncle migrates to the United States from Skidel. He died in 1917
1909	First flight across the English Channel by Louis Blériot
1911	Roald Amundsen reaches the South Pole
1912	U.S. troops occupy Nicaragua (until 1933) Sun Yat-sen becomes president of the new republic of China only to be exiled in 1913
	Birth of Bernard G. Sarnat, Chicago, Illinois
1914	Assassination of Archduke Ferdinand begins World War I (1914–1918) Panama Canal opens
1915	Ethnic cleansing of Armenians by Turkish troops kills 1.3 million Sinking of the Lusitania with a loss of 1,198 lives

General Theory of Relativity published by Albert Einstein

First transcontinental phone call by Alexander Graham Bell

	Birth of Rhoda Gerard in Chicago, Illinois, Bernie's future wife

1917   Collapse of the Russian Tsarist government and the beginning of Russian revolution leading to control by the Bolsheviks

U.S. under Woodrow Wilson enters World War I

	Bernie enters Kindergarten at von Humboldt School

1918   Flu pandemic kills 20–30 million worldwide

	Bernie's family moves to 2558 West Iowa Street
	Bernie enters second grade at Chopin Elementary School
	Bernie's father becomes a naturalized citizen

1920   Prohibition begins (lasts until 1933)

	Bernie's parents buy a building at 3236 Evergreen Avenue
	Bernie begins fourth grade at Lowell Grammar School

Irish Republican Army (IRA) formed

American women are given the vote

1921   Isadore buys his brother-in-law's general store (sells it in 1922)

	Bernie at age nine had a paper route

1922   Soviet Union formed with Joseph Stalin as general secretary

Italian Fascists begin takeover with Benito Mussolini as prime minister

1923	Adolf Hitler imprisoned after failed attempt to seize power in Munich

Bernie's father purchases drugstore at 65th and Blackstone Avenue

Bernie's family moves to 1449 East 66th Place

Bernie enters 5th grade at Walter Scott elementary school at 64th and Blackstone

1924	Vladimir Lenin, architect of the Russian Revolution, dies

Bernie joins the Boys Scouts at age twelve

1925	Joseph Stalin emerges as the ruler of the Soviet Union
1926	Hirohito becomes emperor of Japan

Bernie starts Hyde Park High School (attends 1926–1929)

Bernie attends his first Boy Scout summer camp

Bernie's father loses lease of first drugstore and starts a second one at 69th and Indiana Avenue

Bernie's family moves (again) to an apartment at 7019 Michigan Avenue

1927	Charles Lindbergh makes first non-stop flight across Atlantic Al Jolson stars in The Jazz Singer, the first talking motion picture
1928	Chiang Kai-shek elected president of China President Herbert Hoover wins election Alexander Fleming discovers penicillin
1929	Massacre of 200+ Jews by Palestinians in Hebron

Bernie's father sells his second drugstore to his clerk and buys his third and last drugstore at 57th Street and Blackstone Avenue

	Bernie's family moves again to 5521 University Avenue
	Bernie enters the University of Chicago with advanced standing

	Wall Street crash leading to the Great Depression
1931	Japanese troops invade Manchuria

	Bernie's family moves once more to 5527 Dorchester

1932	Franklin Delano Roosevelt wins election, begins New Deal

	Bernie's parents begin building a modest summer home at Paw Paw Lake, Michigan

1933	Adolf Hitler is appointed chancellor of Germany
	U.S. government repeals Prohibition

	Bernie's family moves once more to 1461 East 56th Street
	Bernie graduates from the University of Chicago with a bachelor's degree and enters medical school (1933–1936)

1934	Mao Zedong retreats to the north to escape Nationalist forces in China
1935	Nuremberg Laws deprive Jews of their citizenship rights
	Italian troops invade Abyssinia
1936	Edward VIII abdicates and George VI takes the throne
	German troops reoccupy the Rhineland in defiance of the 1919 treaty of Versailles
	Spanish Civil War begins (ends 1939)
	Olympics held in Berlin
	Stalin holds show trials of his opponents in Moscow
	Franklin Delano Roosevelt wins re-election

	Bernie graduates from medical school
	Bernie drives to Los Angeles for a year of medical internship

1937	Arab and Jewish communities fight each other over Jewish migration into Palestine The Hindenburg, a German-built airship, explodes at Lakehurst, New Jersey Japanese troops commit "Rape of Nanking" with 250,000 Chinese killed Golden Gate Bridge in San Francisco, the world's longest suspension bridge at that time, is completed

	Bernie returns to Chicago to start his dental and graduate degrees at the University of Illinois (1937–1940)

1938	Adolf Hitler annexes (Anschluss) his native Austria to Germany The German army completes its occupation of the Sudetenland Kristallnacht (Night of Broken Glass), Nazi pogrom — against Jews in Germany Japanese troops occupy most of China, including Peking (Beijing)

	Bernie joins the Army Medical Reserve Corps as first lieutenant

1939	German troops march into Prague and annex Czechoslovakia End of Spanish Civil War with Francisco Franco as dictator Germany invades Poland, starting World War II

	Bernie signs up as ship's doctor for the Cleveland and Buffalo Steamship Company (summers of 1939, 1940 and 1941)

1940   Germany invades The Netherlands, Belgium and Luxembourg
Allied troops are evacuated from Dunkirk to Britain
France surrenders to Germany
Battle of Britain
Franklin Delano Roosevelt is elected to third term

	Bernie awarded coveted Capps prize for research by the Institute of Medicine of Chicago
	Bernie is awarded M.S. and D.D.S. degrees
	Bernie starts a year's residency in Oral and Plastic Surgery

1941   Congress passes the Lend-Lease Act to aid Britain
German troops invade the Soviet Union in Operation Barbarossa
Attack on Pearl Harbor leads to the entrance of the U.S. into World War II

	Bernie marries Rhoda on December 25th, 1941

1942   The extermination of European Jews is planned at the Wannsee
Conference in Berlin
Japanese troops capture Singapore
American troops defeat the Japanese fleet in the Battle of Midway
British troops beat the German army at El Alamein in North Africa
Soviet troops begin a counteroffensive against German army at Stalingrad
Manhattan Project started to develop an atom bomb

German scientists build the V1 and V2 rocket bombs

Bernie is called up for active duty, but did not pass the physical exam

Bernie continues his education with an Assistantship in General Surgery

1943   300,000 German troops surrender at Stalingrad
Allied troops invade Sicily, leads to the fall of Benito Mussolini
Soviet troops win the Battle of Kursk
Tehran Conference, involving Roosevelt, Churchill and Stalin

Assistantship in General Plastic and Reconstructive Surgery in St. Louis

1944   Rome is liberated by Allied troops
D-Day invasion of German-occupied France by Allied troops
Plot by German officers to assassinate Adolf Hitler fails
Battle of Leyte Gulf in the Philippines
Paris is liberated by Allied troops
Franklin Roosevelt wins a fourth term as US president

1945   Yalta Conference involving Churchill, Stalin and an ailing Roosevelt
U.S. president Franklin Roosevelt dies; Harry Truman becomes President
Benito Mussolini and his mistress are shot by Italian partisans
Adolf Hitler marries Eva Braun and both commit suicide in Berlin
Germany surrenders and is divided into Soviet, American, British and French occupation zones
U.S. aircraft drop atomic bombs on Hiroshima and Nagasaki

On the order of Emperor Hirohito, Japan surrenders, ending World War II

Military Tribunal in Nuremberg finds Nazi leaders guilty and issues death penalty verdicts to twelve of them (carried out in 1946)

Bernie's and Rhoda's first child, Gerard, born in St. Louis

1946 Civil war starts between Communist and Nationalist Chinese (ends in 1949)

Military Tribunal in Tokyo finds Prime Minister Hideki Tojo and six others guilty and are sentenced to death

Bernie and family return to Chicago
Bernie is appointed Professor and Chief of Oral and Plastic Surgery, University of Illinois College of Dentistry

1947 European economic recovery is facilitated with the Marshall Plan

Partition of India and Pakistan (Kashmir remains disputed territory)

1948 State of Israel is formed and almost immediately attacked by forces from Egypt, Jordan, Iraq and Syria

Afrikaner Party wins election in South Africa and soon apartheid laws are in place against blacks

Bernie's and Rhoda's second child, Joan, born in Chicago

1949 North Atlantic Treaty Organization (NATO) is formed

Mao Zedong establishes the People's Republic of China

Germany divided into the democratic Federal Republic of Germany and The German Democratic Republic (Communist) in the East

Chinese Nationalists evacuate to Formosa (now Taiwan)

	Isadore, Bernie's father retires

1950	Senator Joseph McCarthy starts anti-communist witch-hunt North Korean troops invade South Korea (war ends 1953)

	Bernie receives the International Kerbs Award for research in Plastic Surgery

1951	Bernie's parents celebrate their 50th wedding anniversary

	Bernie's mother dies quite suddenly from a coronary at age 71

1952	Dwight D. Eisenhower wins victory in the U.S. presidential election
1953	Josef Stalin dies in the Soviet Union
1954	Gamal Abdel Nasser becomes prime minister of Egypt The polio vaccine, developed by Dr. Jonas Salk (1952), now in wide use
1955	East European Communist countries form the Warsaw Pact

	Bernie resigns his University of Illinois appointments and terminates his private practice

	Bernie, Rhoda, Gerard and Joan move permanently to Beverly Hills

1956	Soviet leader Nikita Khrushchev denounces Stalin's crimes Gamal Abdel Nasser is elected president of Egypt, nationalizes the Suez Canal instigating the Suez crisis Soviet troops suppress the popular Hungarian uprising Dwight D. Eisenhower wins re-election Cuban revolution under Fidel Castro initiated

	Bernie's family moves into 616 North Maple Drive, Beverly Hills

	Bernie starts his private practice in Beverly Hills

1957   Sputnik satellites into orbit by the Soviet Union and the space race begins

> Bernie receives senior International Research Award in Plastic Surgery

1959   Fidel Castro enters Havana and proclaims himself prime minister

1960   Israel announces the arrest of Adolf Eichmann (executed in 1962)

John F. Kennedy is elected 35th president

1961   Bay of Pigs invasion in Cuba, which fails

The Berlin Wall is built to keep people from traveling to the west

> Bernie's bout with cancer of the bowel

1962   Cuban missile crisis eventually resolved when Soviet leader, Nikita

Krushchev backs down

1963   President John F. Kennedy is assassinated in Dallas

> Rhoda's mother, Florence, dies at age 88

1964   Palestinian Liberation Organization (PLO) is formed in Jordan

The Gulf of Tonkin incident is used to escalate the war in Vietnam

Nikita Khrushchev is replaced by Leonid Brezhnev

Lyndon Johnson wins the presidency over Barry Goldwater

> Bernie's father, Isadore Sarnat, dies at age 86

1965   Winston Churchill dies

U.S. Marines arrive in Vietnam as the Vietnam War intensifies (ends 1975)

Major race riots break out in the Watts neighborhood of Los Angeles

1966	Mao Zedong publishes his Little Red Book and begins the Cultural Revolution

> Bernie's 25th anniversary party held at 616 North Maple Drive

1967	Israel defeats Egypt, Jordan and Syria in the Six-Day War Dr. Christiaan Barnard performs the first heart transplant in South Africa

> Bernie's appointment in the Section of Oral Biology, UCLA School of Dentistry

	Argentinean/Cuban revolutionary Che Guevara is executed in Bolivia
1968	The "Prague Spring" is brutally suppressed by Soviet tanks North Vietnamese Tet offensive against South Vietnamese cities Dr. Martin Luther King is assassinated in Memphis, Tennessee French students and workers strike, bringing France to a standstill Robert Kennedy, brother of JFK, is assassinated in Los Angeles Richard Nixon is elected 37th president of the United States
1969	Yasser Arafat is elected chairman of the PLO Astronaut Neil Armstrong becomes the first to set foot on the surface of the moon
1971	Idi Amin overthrows Milton Obote of Uganda and becomes dictator War breaks out between East and West Pakistan, which leads to an independent Bangladesh (the former East Pakistan)
1972	At the Olympics in Munich, West Germany, 11 Israeli athletes are massacred by Black September Palestinian terrorists

U.S. President Nixon is re-elected

> Bernie made honorary member of the International Association for the study of Dental Facial Abnormalities

1973   All parties sign the Paris Agreement leading to a cease-fire in Vietnam

Last US troops leave Vietnam

Watergate hearings begin in Washington D.C.

Egypt and Syria invade Israel; the Yom Kippur War begins

1974   U.S. president Richard Nixon resigns after complicity in the cover-up of the burglary at the Watergate democratic headquarters

1975   North Vietnamese troops capture Saigon uniting Vietnam

Microsoft co-founded by the 19-year-old Bill Gates

1976   Mao Zedong dies in Beijing

Democrat Jimmy Carter wins the U.S. presidential election

1977   Egyptian President Anwar Sadat pays a surprise visit to Israel

1978   Camp David accords between Jimmy Carter, Menachem Begin and Anwar Sadat

1979   Shah of Iran flees and Ayatollah Khomeini returns to lead the government

The Idi Amin regime is overthrown by Tanzanian troops

Saddam Hussein becomes president of Iraq

Soviet troops invade Afghanistan, and a 10-year war begins

1980   Iraq invades Iran (war ends 1988)

Ronald Reagan becomes the 40th president

> Bernie receives Cottle Award from the American Rhinologic Society

1981   Prince Charles marries Lady Diana Spencer

Egypt's President Anwar Sadat is assassinated by Islamic fundamentalists

	CDC recognizes acquired immune deficiency syndrome (Aids)
1982	Falklands War between Britain and Argentina begins
1984	Ronald Reagan is re-elected U.S. president
1985	Mikhail Gorbachev advocates "glasnost" and "perestroika"
1986	U.S. space shuttle Challenger explodes on take-off, killing all its crew
	Iran-Contra scandal implicates the Ronald Reagan's presidency
1987	Palestinians begin an intifada (uprising) against Israeli rule
	Chinese troops suppress a nationalist uprising in Tibet

> Bernie receives the Distinguished Alumni Service Award from the University of Chicago Pritzler School of Medicine

1988	Soviet troops begin to withdraw from Afghanistan
	A ceasefire ends the Iran-Iraq War
	George H. W. Bush wins victory for U.S. president

> Bernie receives the International Alpha Omega Award

1989	East Germany opens its borders and the Berlin Wall is pulled down
	Václav Havel is elected Czechoslovakia's president
	Romanian dictator Nicolae Ceausescu and his wife Elena are executed
1990	Nelson Mandela is released from prison after 27 years
	Boris Yeltsin is elected president of the Russian Federation
	Iraqi troops invade Kuwait, beginning the Gulf War (ends 1991)
	Lech Walesa is elected president of Poland

> Bernie receives the International Honorary Award from the American Society of Maxillofacial Surgeons

1991   Coalition forces liberate Kuwait. Saddam Hussein is
        defeated, but remains in power
        Apartheid ends in South Africa
        Civil war begins in the former Yugoslavia
        Soviet Union officially ceases to exist

Bernie retires from surgical practice

1992   William Jefferson 'Bill' Clinton, wins the U.S. presi-
        dential election
        Deng Xiaoping supports free-market economics

For Bernie's and Rhoda's 50th anniversary; the family went on a Mexican cruise

1993   Czechoslovakia becomes two countries: the Slovak
        Republic (Slovakia) and the Czech Republic

Bernie made an Honorary Fellow of the American Association of Plastic Surgeons

1994   Nelson Mandela is elected the first black president of
        South Africa
        Irish Republican Army (IRA) announces a complete
        cessation of violence
        Russian troops invade the breakaway republic of
        Chechnya
1995   Israeli Prime Minister Yitzhak Rabin is assassinated

Bernie receives the International Craniofacial Biology Research Award from the International Association for Dental Research (IADR)

1996   In Russia, Boris Yeltsin is re-elected president
        U.S. president Bill Clinton wins re-election
1997   Chinese leader Deng Xiaoping dies, aged 92
        Britain returns Hong Kong to China, and peaceful
        reunification occurs
        Britain's Princess Diana dies in a car crash in Paris
        Taliban troops capture Kabul in Afghanistan

1999	General Pervez Musharraf overthrows Pakistan's government
	Russian president Boris Yeltsin resigns, his successor is Vladimir Putin

	Bernie receives the Pioneer in Medicine Award from the Cedars-Sinai Medical Center, Los Angeles

2000	George W. Bush becomes president in a bitterly contested election
2002	President Bush unilaterally invades and occupies Iraq

2003	Bernie received the University of Chicago Alumni At Large Award

2004	George W. Bush re-elected for a second term by a narrow margin

2004	Bernie receives the University of Illinois in Chicago Alumni Achievement Award

2005	Bernie's 93rd birthday celebration

2006	Elections return control to Democrats in Congress

CONFERRED HONORS

1940   Joseph A. Capps Prize (co-winner) for Medical Research offered by the Institute of Medicine of Chicago, Illinois (Chicago)

1950   J.E. Kerbs Junior Award, international competition for original research in Plastic Surgery offered by the Foundation of the American Society of Plastic and Reconstructive Surgeons (Mexico City)

1957   Senior Award, international competition for original research in Plastic Surgery offered by the Foundation of the American Society of Plastic and Reconstructive Surgeons (San Francisco)

1958   Beverly Hills Academy of Medicine Award (Beverly Hills, CA)

1964   Phi Epsilon Pi National Achievement Award (Medicine) (Los Angeles)

1972   Honorary Member, International Association for the study of Dental Facial Abnormalities

1980   Cottle Award from the American Rhinologic Society

1980   Dedication in Laskin's text of Oral and Maxillofacial Surgery (C.V. Mosby, Pub.)

1985   Medal, Tel Aviv University, Tel Aviv, Israel (Tel Aviv)

1985   Medal, Hebrew University, Jerusalem, Israel (Jerusalem)

1987   Distinguished Service Alumni Award, University of Chicago Pritzker School of Medicine. The Distinguished

Service Awards recognize alumni who, by demonstrating outstanding leadership in and making significant contributions to the health field through basic research, clinical care, health service administration, or public service/civic duties have brought honor and distinction to the Medical School and to the University of Chicago (Chicago)

1988   International Alpha Omega Achievement Medal for outstanding contributions to the fields of Dentistry and Plastic and Reconstructive Surgery (Fort Lauderdale)

1990   International Honorary Award, American Society of Maxillofacial Surgeons (Boston)

1993   Honorary Fellow, American Association of Plastic Surgeons. This Award is given for outstanding contributions in the areas of education, research or clinical excellence based on a life-long career (Philadelphia)

1993   Dallas B. Phemister Professional Achievement Award. Department of Surgery, the University of Chicago in recognition of lifetime distinction in the field of plastic surgery (San Francisco)

1994   Distinguished Alumni Award, University of Illinois College of Dentistry (In absentia)

1994   UCLA Division of Plastic Surgery (San Diego)

1995   Distinguished Scientist International IADR Craniofacial Biology Research Award (Singapore)

1999   Pioneer in Medicine Award. Cedars-Sinai Medical Center Staff (Los Angeles). Internationally recognized for more than five decades as a Pioneer Craniofacial Biologist, Plastic and Reconstructive Surgeon, Researcher and Educator

2000   Honorary Member, American Association of Pediatric Plastic Surgeons (Los Angeles)

2003   Professional Achievement Citation to recognize alumni who have brought distinction to themselves, credit to the University and benefit to their communities through their vocational work, University of Chicago Alumni Association (Chicago)

2003   Citation of Excellence in Research (First Awardee), Plastic Surgery Educational Foundation (San Diego)

2004   University of Illinois in Chicago Alumni Achievement Award is the highest honor bestowed by the Alumni Association on behalf of the University. It is presented to an alumnus who has attained outstanding success and national or international distinction in his profession, and whose accomplishments bring honor to the University (Chicago)

2004   American Society of Maxillofacial Surgeons Honorary Member for his service, dedication and commitment to the field of maxillofacial and craniofacial surgery

2005   Best Paper of the Year 2004 (Intersitial Growth of Bone Revisited) in the Journal of Craniofacial Surgery

2006   Dedication in Laskin's text Temporomandibular Disorders (Quintessence Pub.)

2007   Honorary Faculty Marshal at UCLA David Geffen School of Medicine Graduation

AVAILABLE ADDITIONAL INFORMATION
ON BERNARD G. SARNAT

[1] National Archives of Plastic Surgery:
Francis A. Countway, Library of Medicine, Harvard Medical School
10 Shattuck Street, Boston, MA 02115
617-732-2173; 617-432-4142

[2] Archives of the University of California at Los Angeles:
Charlotte B. Brown
21560 Young Research Library
310-825-7265